The Complete Idiot's Reference Card

Common Running Distances

400 meters: One lap around an outdoor track. Four laps equals one mile.

Kilometer: The metric standard used internationally to measure races. One kilometer equals .621 miles.

5K: The most popular distance for road races. 5K equals 3.1 miles.

10K: The second most popular distance for road races. 10K equals 6.2 miles.

Marathon: The crown jewel of running. A marathon is 26.2 miles long (26 miles, 385 yards).

Quick Pace Guide

1 mile	2 miles	5K	5 miles	10K	Marathon
7:00	14:00	21:45	35:00	43:30	3:03:03
7:30	15:00	23:18	37:30	46:36	3:16:39
8:00	16:00	24:51	40:00	49:42	3:29:45
8:30	17:00	26:24	42:30	52:48	3:42:51
9:00	18:00	27:57	45:00	55:54	3:56:00
9:30	19:00	29:30	47:30	59:00	4:09:03
10:00	20:00	31:03	50:00	1:02:06	4:22:12
10:30	21:00	32:36	52:30	1:05:12	4:35:19
11:00	22:00	34:09	55:00	1:08:18	4:48:24
11:30	23:00	35:42	57:30	1:11:24	5:01:30
12:00	24:00	37:15	1:00:00	1:15:30	5:14:38

alpha
books

Essential Stretches for Runners

- ➤ Foot/ankle stretch
- ➤ Achilles tendon/calves stretch
- ➤ Hamstring stretch
- ➤ Iliotibial band stretch

- ➤ Hips/butt stretch
- ➤ Groin stretch
- ➤ Back stretch

Talk the Talk

aerobic exercise   Exercise such as running that you do for at least 20 minutes at a comfortable pace.

biomechanics   How your body parts work together to create your running form.

carboloading   Eating extra carbohydrates in the few days before a long race to have more stored fuel during the race. It's only necessary in races that take more than an hour to complete.

DNF   Stands for "did not finish" a race.

fartlek   A Swedish term for "speed play." It's doing speed work in an unstructured way on roads or trails.

intervals   Doing speed work on a track. You run fast for a specified distance, run slowly for a specified time or distance to recover, and then repeat the process a specified number of times.

long run   A run done about once a week that's at least one and a half times longer than any other run in that week.

orthotics   Devices put in shoes to improve runners' biomechanics and lower their injury risk.

overpronation   When your feet roll in too much after your heel hits the ground when you run. It's one of the leading causes of injury to runners.

PR   Stands for "personal record," which is your best performance at a certain distance.

speed work   Running a workout of several runs of a mile or shorter at race pace or faster, with slow recovery jogs between the hard runs.

splits   Intermediate times en route to a longer distance, such as mile times in a 5K.

tapering   Cutting back on running soon before a big race to conserve your energy.

The Wall   What you crash into if you run out of energy in a marathon. For most runners, that happens after about 20 miles, but with the right training, pre-race nutrition, and race pace, you can avoid it.

THE COMPLETE IDIOT'S GUIDE® TO

Jogging and Running

by Bill Rodgers
with Scott Douglas

alpha books

A Division of Macmillan General Reference
A Simon & Schuster Macmillan Company
1633 Broadway, New York, NY 10019-6785

©1998 by Bill Rodgers

All rights reserved. No part of this book shall be reproduced, stored in a retrieval system, or transmitted by any means, electronic, mechanical, photocopying, recording, or otherwise, without written permission from the publisher. No patent liability is assumed with respect to the use of the information contained herein. Although every precaution has been taken in the preparation of this book, the publisher and author assume no responsibility for errors or omissions. Neither is any liability assumed for damages resulting from the use of information contained herein. For information, address Alpha Books, 1633 Broadway, 7th Floor, New York, NY 10019-6785.

THE COMPLETE IDIOT'S GUIDE TO Design is a registered trademark of Prentice-Hall, Inc.

Macmillan Publishing books may be purchased for business or sales promotional use. For information please write: Special Markets Department, Macmillan Publishing USA, 1633 Broadway, New York, NY 10019.

International Standard Book Number: 0-02-862386-X
Library of Congress Catalog Card Number: 98-84950

00 99 98   8 7 6 5 4 3 2

Interpretation of the printing code: the rightmost number of the first series of numbers is the year of the book's printing; the rightmost number of the second series of numbers is the number of the book's printing. For example, a printing code of 98-1 shows that the first printing occurred in 1998.

Printed in the United States of America

Note: This publication contains the opinions and ideas of its author. It is intended to provide helpful and informative material on the subject matter covered. It is sold with the understanding that the author and publisher are not engaged in rendering professional services in the book. If the reader requires personal assistance or advice, a competent professional should be consulted.

The author and publisher specifically disclaim any responsibility for any liability, loss or risk, personal or otherwise, which is incurred as a consequence, directly or indirectly, of the use and application of any of the contents of this book.

ALPHA DEVELOPMENT TEAM

Publisher
Kathy Nebenhaus

Editorial Director
Gary M. Krebs

Managing Editor
Bob Shuman

Marketing Brand Manager
Felice Primeau

Senior Editor
Nancy Mikhail

Development Editors
Phil Kitchel
Jennifer Perillo
Amy Zavatto

Editorial Assistant
Maureen Horn

PRODUCTION TEAM

Development Editor
Nader Mikhail

Production Editor
Mark Enochs

Copy Editor
Heather Stith

Cover Designer
Mike Freeland

Photo Editor
Richard H. Fox

Photography
Stacey Cramp

Illustrator
Jody P. Schaeffer

Designer
Glenn Larsen

Indexer
Chris Barrick

Layout/Proofreading
Angela Calvert
Kim Cofer
Mary Hunt

Contents at a Glance

14.36

Contents

vii

Foreword

It should come as no surprise to readers of this book that Bill Rodgers has chosen to author *The Complete Idiot's Guide to Jogging and Running*. After all, only an idiot would attempt to run as many miles as Bill has run during his remarkable career. Though Bill has set many records and established many firsts during his career, I would not recommend that any of our readers try to match the miles Bill puts in each week.

Bill has set the pace for American distance running since winning his first Boston Marathon in 1975. Since that time, he went on to win the Boston Marathon three more times and was winner of the New York City Marathon four times. Bill's extensive knowledge of jogging and running is based on his first-hand running experiences, and when coupled with his love for the sport and respect for other runners of all abilities, he clearly stands as the most logical candidate to author *The Complete Idiot's Guide to Jogging and Running*. I know of no other personality in the sport of running who communicates with other runners as effectively as Bill. His popularity as a runner is easy to understand once a person has the opportunity to witness the passion and patience that he displays when talking with other runners. That passion comes shining through in these pages.

The Complete Idiot's Guide to Jogging and Running is a most comprehensive "How to" book. It covers myriad topics relating to running—from tips and techniques on getting started, to more advanced methods of training to be a better runner. The smart chapter and section titles entertain while they inform. This book gives beginners the edge they need to come up with a running plan that works and to help them run competitively.

Since meeting Bill Rodgers over 20 years ago at a half-marathon in Portland, Maine, my running has been enhanced and my life enriched. The personal attention that Bill gave to me after my performance that day inspired me to seriously pursue my running career while setting goals every step of the way. But the most important thing I've learned from Bill is how to give back to the sport that has given us so much. Bill does exactly that in *The Complete Idiot's Guide to Jogging and Running* by sharing valuable information for "idiots" and "non-idiots" alike. His stories and experiences are always entertaining and inspiring. Enjoy the book and then head to the track!

—Joan Benoit Samuelson

Gold medalist, 1984 Olympic Marathon
American record holder in the marathon

Introduction

Ask a group of regular runners if they hope to run for the rest of their lives, and they'll all tell you yes. Me? I've been a runner for more than 30 years, and I hope to still be one 30 years from now.

Running is great exercise—in fact, it's one of the simplest, most effective, and most convenient forms of exercise around. Keep running, and you'll do some incredible things for your health. But running is also a way of life. It's about having more energy, feeling good about yourself, making new friends, challenging yourself, enjoying nature, and a million other things that I want to tell you about. As you might have guessed, I love running. In this book, I hope to pass on that passion to you.

How to Use This Book

This book is divided into five parts. Think of them as five different runs, all interesting and enjoyable enough on their own, but even more so when combined with the others.

Part 1, "In the Beginning," tells you what you need to know to start a running program. I'll explain why so many people run and how running helps your health. I'll give you a training plan that will take you from no running to 30 minutes at a time in just a month. Also, I'll give you tips about how to find the time to run, where to run, and how to stay motivated.

Part 2, "The Right Stuff," deals with the main equipment that runners use. The most important thing here is a good pair of running shoes. I'll show you how to pick a pair that's right for you. I'll also list what running apparel you need to run comfortably. And I'll highlight some of the best running gadgets. At the end of this section, you'll know how to look the part.

Part 3, "Body Shop," is all about the most important part of your running—your body. I'll show you how to prevent injuries with the right stretching and strengthening exercises. I'll also tell you how to treat common injuries, describe the runners' diet, highlight what's special about running for women, and explain how to run comfortably in different kinds of weather. Your legs will thank you once you're armed with this info.

Part 4, "Join the Human Race," deals with my favorite aspect of this sport—racing. I'll explain why racing is so much fun and how to prepare for everything from your local 5K to the marathon and all distances in between.

Part 5, "Running Through the Ages" has special advice for younger and older runners. Regardless of how old you are now, it tells you how to stay a runner for the rest of your life. Isn't that what it's all about?

Extras

Every chapter in this book contains helpful and informative sidebars that show you how to run better and understand running a little bit more:

Footnotes

You never know when someone might ask you who won the Boston Marathon in 1975 (yes, it was Bill Rodgers). These sidebars include bits of running lore, running history, and running facts and figures.

Training Tip

The information in this box is a tidbit of how-to knowledge. Follow the advice here to supplement your running knowledge and training.

Rules of the Road

It takes more than proper form and training to become a good runner. These sidebars teach you about running safety and etiquette for when you're ready to put your best feet forward.

Track Talk

What is a split, DNF, and fartlek? Look for these sidebars to learn today's running lingo.

Acknowledgments

Although running is primarily an individual sport, you need the support and guidance of family and friends, coaches, and training partners to do your best. So thanks most of all to my parents, my brother Charlie, and sisters Linda and Martha for all of their support over the years, as well as to my wife, Gail, for her understanding help as I've continued to aim for excellence in competitive running.

For showing me how to stay on the road, sincere thanks to Frank O'Rourke, who guided my best friend, Jason Kehoe, Charlie, and me through our first year of running in 1963. He must have done something right, because we're all still at it! My Wesleyan University coach, Elmer Swanson, taught me commitment and how to keep running fun, and Billy Squires, America's finest marathon coach, guided me and many others to the top of the marathon world.

Thanks also to my co-author, Scott Douglas, for joining me and successfully completing this marathon challenge; to photographer Stacey Cramp, who worked quickly and smoothly to make me look good; and to the folks at Athletic Express in Gaithersburg, Maryland, for the use of their fine facility for our photos.

Special Thanks from the Publisher to the Technical Reviewer

The Complete Idiot's Guide to Jogging and Running was reviewed by an expert who not only checked the technical accuracy of what you'll learn in this book, but also provided invaluable insight and suggestions to ensure that you learn everything you need to know when deciding on starting a running program. Our special thanks are extended to **Jim Hage**, contributing editor to *Running Times* magazine, road racing correspondent for *The Washington Post,* and host of "Jim Hage's Running Report" on WMAL AM 630 radio in Washington, DC. He won the Marine Corps Marathon in 1988 and 1989 and finished eighth in the 1992 Olympic Trials Marathon.

Part 1
In the Beginning

Everywhere you look these days, you see runners. Your neighbor is a runner. Your co-worker is a runner. Heck, President Clinton is a runner, and Vice President Gore has run a marathon. So has Oprah Winfrey. What's going on? What's so great about running?

In the first part of this book, I'll tell you some of the million reasons why people run. You'll learn that running gives you more energy, helps you lose weight, and allows you to reclaim your youth, among other things. If you've always used the "I don't have the time" excuse, I'll show you how you can fit running into your busy life and still be gainfully employed. Once I've got you going, I'll do my part to keep you going with special motivational strategies that long-time runners use.

Chapter 1

Hit the Road, Jack and Jill

In This Chapter

➤ Why to start running

➤ How many runners there are in the United States

➤ The kinder, gentler face of running in the '90s

➤ The difference between running and jogging

➤ Common myths about running

Twenty-five years ago, when I started training seriously for marathons, most people who saw someone running down the street thought that person was either a crook or a kook. That's no longer the case. During the last two decades, running has become a regular part of American life. Three of the last four Presidents have been runners, and the current Vice President, Al Gore, finished a marathon in the fall of 1997. Most people now know that running a few times a week on a regular basis is one of the best things you can do to take control of your health. In this chapter, I'll show you other reasons to start running, as well as give you a sense of how many other runners there are and what they're like so that you'll know whom you'll be sharing the roads with.

Reasons to Run

How do I love running? Let me count the ways. There are as many reasons to run as there are runners, and that's a lot of reasons! Most people, of course, run for physical reasons (or at least that's why they start to run); they want to lose weight, fight a family history of heart disease, or just feel better.

Other people run for different reasons. A lot of runners, especially young ones, get into it for the competition. They want to see how fast they can run a mile or whether they can beat their next-door neighbor in the local 5K. Other people run primarily for psychological reasons. They like the stress relief, reflection time, and sense of being in control that running brings.

Here's a baker's dozen of some of the most popular reasons to run:

1. Running is a great way to lose weight.
2. Regular *aerobic exercise*, such as running, decreases the risk of heart disease.
3. Running is one of the most effective ways to improve *cardiovascular fitness*.
4. Running is a great way to quit smoking.
5. Regular aerobic exercise reduces the risk of some cancers.
6. When you become fitter by running, you're more likely to improve other aspects of your lifestyle, such as your diet.
7. Running is the most convenient of sports; you can do it almost anytime, anywhere.
8. People who have a high level of physical fitness usually have a positive self-image.
9. Running is cheap; all you need are a good pair of running shoes and a few pieces of running apparel.

Track Talk

Aerobic exercise means working out at a moderate level so that you're not out of breath for at least 20 minutes at a time. *Aerobic* means "with oxygen;" examples of aerobic exercises are distance running, swimming, cycling, and walking.

10. Fitter people are more productive on the job.
11. Running with others is a great way to build friendships.
12. Being fit increases mental sharpness; regular exercisers are able to concentrate longer and are better problem solvers.
13. Running is one of the best stress relievers around.

You might have noticed that some of these reasons can apply to other forms of exercise, such as cycling or walking. I have nothing against these sports, but you might have also noticed that some of these reasons only pertain to running.

The combination of what running has in common with other ways to work out and its unique features is what, in my humble opinion, makes it the best exercise choice for the greatest number of people. You might not believe me now, but here are two more important reasons to run that you'll discover if you stick with it for just a bit: Running feels good while you're doing it and after you've done it, and it's tons of fun!

The next chapter looks in depth at how running helps to improve your health. I'm guessing that if you've picked up this book, you already know about some of running's health benefits and that those all-important health reasons are among your strongest reasons for having an interest in running. So indulge me a bit here while I go off on a slightly different tack and tell you a little bit about why I started running. My point in doing so is to show you that, like you probably do, I had a lot of different motivations. One of the great things about running is that with so many compelling reasons to do it, these reasons tend to reinforce each other (at least that was the case with me).

Like a lot of kids, I started running as a member of a high school team. I ran a one-mile race put on by the Newington, CT Parks and Recreation Department when I was in my mid teens. I was able to win in a time of 5:20. I liked being good at something (and being better than the other kids), so I went out for the high school cross-country and track teams. I won the state championship in cross-country, and I got my mile time down to 4:28. I was drawn to running as a racer, but I also discovered that I simply liked to run. I liked how it felt when I did it. I liked the sense of being outside and exploring nature with my friends on the team. People usually don't think of these reasons for running right off the bat.

One of my goals in college had been to break 9:00 for two miles, and I achieved it. But when I got out of college in 1970, I stopped running. With so much else going on in my life at the time, I figured, what was the point of continuing to run? I drifted for a couple of years, working menial jobs to fulfill the requirements of being a conscientious objector. I started drinking a little too much, a little too often. And I became a smoker.

> **Track Talk**
> *Cardiovascular fitness* is the ability to sustain comfortably a moderate level of aerobic exercise. It's what people mean when they talk about stamina or endurance—being fit enough to keep up a decent level of activity. Of the main components of fitness, cardiovascular fitness is the most important and directly relates to your risk of heart disease and some cancers.

> **Track Talk**
> A *marathon* is a race that's 26 miles, 385 yards long. It's the farthest that most runners ever go. It's not accurate to call any long race a marathon because the name refers to the specific distance of 26.2 miles.

In 1972, Frank Shorter, an American, won the Olympic *Marathon*. I didn't know Frank then, but he's my age. I remember watching him win that race on television. Something in the back of my mind tugged at me to become a runner again.

I can recall from around this time sitting in a bar and thinking, "This can't be it. This just can't be it. There has to be something more to life than drinking and smoking." Gradually, in fits and starts, I started to run again, for a whole new set of reasons. Competition wasn't my driving goal. Something more important was taking control of my life. When I was at my depths, running gave me back my self-esteem.

Training Tip
If you're trying to quit smoking, one of the best ways to fight the urge to light up is to get outside and move around for a bit. The fresh air makes all that tar and nicotine that much more distasteful. I used this method to kick my two-pack-a-day habit.

Running helped me to quit smoking, because as I became fitter, smoking became that much less enjoyable. Eventually, I got excited about competition again and ran the first race of my comeback in 1973. Two years later, I won the first of four Boston Marathons.

Why am I telling you all this? Because I want you to see that every runner, even someone like me who you might think was born running a million miles a day at an ungodly speed, was at some point a confused, unsure beginner. But, like me, every runner also soon discovers his or her own endless reasons for sticking with it. Ask any group of regular runners if they want to run for the rest of their lives, and the answer will be a unanimous yes. That is perhaps the single best reason to run: When you're a runner, life is better.

8,000,000 Runners Can't Be Wrong

How many runners are there in the United States? That depends on who you ask and who you define as a runner. According to the National Sporting Goods Association (NSGA), more than 22 million Americans ran in 1996. That's about one in 12 Americans! However, the NSGA figures count anyone who ran more than five times that year as a runner. So that statistic includes all those people who made a New Year's resolution to run, hit the roads a few times a week for a month, but then gave it up as they lost motivation (does this describe you?).

I'm not saying that it's not great that 22 million Americans ran more than five times in 1996. But running is different from something like camping, which, according to the NSGA, more than 44 million Americans did in 1996. The hard-core outdoorsy crowd might not agree with me here, but if you go camping once a month or so, you can safely say that you're a camper.

Running is different. Within even a week of training, your cardiovascular fitness starts to improve. Unfortunately, the reverse is also true—stop running, and you start to lose the benefits. If you run 10 times in a month and then give it up for six months, you'll be starting from scratch if you take it up again. Contrast that with camping, where you might take a few trips in the summer and then not go again until spring. I'd bet you wouldn't find yourself just standing at the campsite, baffled as to how to set up a tent, start a fire, and so on.

To be a runner, you have to keep at it. That's why the statistics gathered by American Sports Data (ASD), a research organization that tracks Americans' participation in 58 sports and activities, provide more accurate numbers. In addition to overall participation, this organization tracks what it calls "frequent participation." For running, frequent participation means going at least 100 times in a year. That number seems right to me. If you run at least 100 times per year, you're probably running about twice a week. That's really the minimum of what you can do and expect to make progress in terms of endurance, distance, and so on.

Just a little more than 8 million Americans met ASD's definition of frequent participants in running in 1996. It's not 22 million, but it's still a lot of people—roughly 3 percent of the American population running at least twice a week. Even more encouraging is the fact that more than 5 million Americans ran at least 150 days in 1996, according to ASD. That's almost every other day. Only fitness walking and lifting with free weights can claim more adherents at this level of participation.

Running in the '90s

Just who are these 8 million runners who are so dedicated that they're out there more than 100 days a year? They're not who you might think they are. When a lot of people think about running, they think about the movie *Rocky*. Never mind that Rocky was a boxer, not a runner. Based on how many times people have sung the *Rocky* theme at me as I run down their streets, you sure wouldn't know it.

I think a lot of people think of Rocky because they've been led to believe that running is all about pain and torturing yourself and getting up at 5 a.m. And they've been led to believe that the only people who run are hard-core competitive athletes training to be among the best in the world. Well, these people need to get a new tune and not just because I never liked that infernal song in the first place.

Unlike a sport such as football, running is a lifetime sport that almost anybody can do. As it turns out, just about anybody *does* do it. More than half of all regular runners are over the age of 40. Nearly half of the 160,000 members of the Road Runners Club of America, the largest national running group, are women. Participation in women-only races increased by 18 percent between 1995 and 1996, more so than for any other type of race. So throw away your image of running being only for that 25-year-old guy down the street who looks as though he could break 4:00 for the mile.

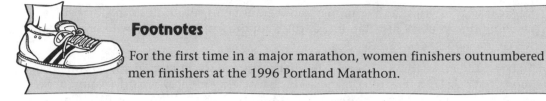

Footnotes

For the first time in a major marathon, women finishers outnumbered men finishers at the 1996 Portland Marathon.

Some of the misconceptions about who runners are stem from the first running boom, which took place in the mid to late 1970s. At that time, a lot of runners were motivated primarily by competition and running high mileage. In some circles, your time for the marathon was the be-all and end-all of your existence. I certainly never thought this way; I've always been for people exploring all that running has to offer and finding the level that they're comfortable with. Yet I'm associated with what some people see as the extremes of the first running boom.

When the boom hit, I was at my peak. I won the Boston Marathon four times between 1975 and 1980. During those years, I also won the New York City Marathon four times. This was just as interest in large-scale running events was taking off. Marathons were held up to be the pinnacle of running achievement.

For a while, running was kind of chic. Even Hunter S. Thompson, the famous "gonzo journalist" for *Rolling Stone*, once covered the Honolulu Marathon. We baby boomers have been pretty good at being the center of the media's attention for most of our lives. During this time, in the late '70s, we were around 30 years old—just about the age at which a marathoner peaks. Getting those peak performances in the marathon requires logging a lot of miles. So in the public's view, running was all about putting in more than 10 miles a day, eating funny, being really thin, and making all these sacrifices to better your time in this strange race called the marathon.

As with most other things, the media eventually got bored with running and moved on to something else. People didn't hear about some of the fundamental changes in running, both in terms of who participates and in their attitudes, for a long time. A lot of those baby boomers who were hard-core marathoners in the first running boom kept right on running. But like everyone else, they had to make adjustments as the years passed. Some of them learned that they just weren't cut out for constant high-mileage training. As their career and family responsibilities increased, their time and energy for running decreased. But the important thing is that most of them kept at it and are still going.

Some people have said that American running is undergoing a second boom, but they say that because the media has started to pay attention again, not because participation numbers have skyrocketed out of nowhere in just the last few years. For example, the number of marathon finishers has been growing steadily for the past several years. In 1996, there were almost 400,000 marathon finishers in the United States. That's about double the number from 1986 and four times as many as in the late '70s, during the supposed "boom."

If there is a second boom going on, what marks it is a difference in participants and their attitudes and motivation. Running in the '90s is said to be kinder and gentler. No longer do you see many people going around trying to flout their status by boasting about their marathon *PR*. The average runner of the '90s runs less than the average runner of the first boom and is drawn to running for health and social reasons more so than for hard-core competition reasons.

But wait a minute. Aren't I contradicting myself by saying that marathon participation has doubled in the last decade, and then saying that running in the '90s is kinder and gentler? No, because even the marathon, which was once taken to be the holy grail of running for which runners had to sacrifice endlessly, is today seen as a solid, but conquerable, challenge for almost any runner.

What that means is that more marathoners are drawn to the event by the challenge of finishing, not seeing how quickly they can do so. "Completing, not competing" is how some people put it. This more relaxed attitude has had the following effect: For 10 marathons held in 1980, 62 percent of the field finished in less than four hours. At those 10 races in 1995, 28.5 percent of the field ran that fast. The median finishing time for men increased by 21 minutes, to 3:54, and for women by 11 minutes, to 4:15.

> **Track Talk**
> *PR* stands for personal record, your best time for a distance. Runners cherish and talk about their PRs the way that new parents talk about their babies.

> **Rules of the Road**
> When you're in the company of other runners, it's common runner's etiquette to talk about your PRs only if you're asked.

> **Footnotes**
> About 60 percent of the 18,000 participants in the 1997 Marine Corps Marathon had never run a marathon before.

Still think that running is only for skinny, fast, always-training competitive athletes? Still think that running isn't embraced by millions of Americans of all ages and shapes and backgrounds as an inclusive, healthful way to lead their lives? Then I'll leave you with this tidbit: In 1994, Oprah Winfrey finished the Marine Corps Marathon. She then appeared on the cover of *Runner's World*. Oprah later said that of all the magazine covers she's ever been on, being on *Runner's World*'s was the biggest thrill. That issue of *Runner's World* is the biggest seller in the magazine's 30-year history.

Footnotes

Runner's World is the most popular running magazine in the world, with a circulation of more than 400,000. The other major American running magazine is *Running Times*.

Running Versus Jogging

What is the difference between jogging and running? There are lots of ways to make the distinction—how far you run, how fast you run, why you run, how often you run, and so on ad infinitum. No, make that ad nauseum. The debates about who's a jogger and who's a runner are endless and fierce, but they're also pointless.

Usually, the distinction is made in a condescending way, with running taken to be superior to jogging. Some runners like to puff themselves up by noting others' speed and saying, "Oh, he's just jogging." Well, we're all slower than someone else. The best runners in the world cover 5 kilometers (3.1 miles; the distance is also called 5K) at just a bit slower than 4:00 per mile. The best marathoners in the world run sub-5:00 miles for 26.2 miles. By their standards, I guess we're all joggers, huh? So let's scratch pace as what makes one person a jogger and another person a runner.

Is the difference the distance run? As I said, about 400,000 Americans completed a marathon in 1996. Bob Kennedy doesn't run farther than 15 miles at a time in his training, but Kennedy holds the American record for 5K, which he has covered at roughly 4:10 per mile. Think any of those marathoners would call him a jogger?

So maybe the difference is how often you run. That has to be good a way to know who's serious (trumpet blasts: a runner!) and who's just dogging it (cue the boos: a jogger). Bob Ray, of Parkville, MD, has run at least 4 miles a day, every day, since April 1968. Ed Eyestone is a Mormon and almost always takes Sunday off from running for religious purposes. Eyestone is also a two-time U.S. Olympian in the marathon. Bob Ray wouldn't call Eyestone a jogger, and neither would anyone else. As you'll see later in this book, it's what you do with your days of running, not how many you can string together, that really matters.

And what about why you run? One old saw is that the difference between a jogger and a runner is an entry form. This saying was supposed to mean that by entering races, you somehow graduated from the vile level of jogger to the promised land of being a runner. I know plenty of people who faithfully put in their miles, but for a variety of reasons choose not to race. One of my old rivals, Tom Fleming, who twice won the New York City Marathon, runs 10 miles most days at faster than 7:00 per mile. But he doesn't care to compete anymore. Does that mean he's now a jogger?

Footnotes

Ron Hill, who won the Boston Marathon in 1970, is generally considered to have the longest running streak (not having missed a day of running) in the world. The last day that Hill didn't run was in 1964.

Another distinction along these lines that I've heard is that joggers are in it for the exercise, runners for the sport. This distinction is just plain silly. I can no more single out the one reason that I run any more than I can name the quality that I love most about my wife. In both cases, many aspects thrill me, and each aspect plays off of all the others.

OK, so what *is* the difference? There isn't any. Jogging, running—call it what you want. You'll know when you're doing more than walking. Why have I spent all this time making this point? Because it's easy for beginning runners to feel that what they're doing isn't important. Often, the people who make them feel that way the most are veteran runners, who forget what it's like to take those first tentative steps. Their attitude can cause a lot of beginners to feel that there's some standard they have to measure up to. There isn't; the only one that matters is your own satisfaction.

Mythical Contortions

While I'm disposing of stale arguments, I'll go ahead and discuss some of the myths you've probably heard about running. Maybe these myths have made you hesitant about starting a running program. Maybe they'll be thrown at you once your Uncle Zeke, that opinionated old cur whom you have to see every Thanksgiving, learns that you've started to run. Whatever the case, the following are a few myths you'll hear about running.

"You never see runners smile."

I guess this statement is supposed to mean that running isn't fun. Apparently, some people think that people should be smiling all the time; to them, if you're not smiling, you're not having a good time. But who would want to live in a world where everyone is always smiling? Sounds too much like *Brave New World*, filled with happy idiots.

More important, these people are just plain wrong. How often do they see runners? Do they see me out running with my friends, talking away for an hour, cracking jokes, telling stories, and sometimes even having to slow down a little because we're laughing so hard? Look around the next time you see people running together. Watch them long enough, and I guarantee you'll see some smiles.

The non-smiling runner Uncle Zeke has seen is probably on a solo run. Where does it say that the only sign of enjoying yourself is a smile? I bet that Uncle Zeke doesn't grin his way through dinner or sex, but he'd probably like to repeat those experiences.

"You'll ruin your knees."

I hear some version of this statement about once a week. I worry more about injuring myself rolling my eyes in reaction than I do about my knees becoming arthritic because of running. Yes, people get injured running. As explained in Chapter 12, however, most of those injuries are predictable and preventable. They're usually caused by trying to do too much too soon at too quick a pace and by ignoring the body's warning signs.

What the ruin-your-knees naysayers usually mean is that running is going to do long-term damage to your body, especially in the form of arthritis. I don't mean to be mean here, and I know that this statement is often made with good intentions, but did you ever notice that the people making it don't exactly look like they view their bodies as temples? Instead, they're using the myth about ruining your knees to justify their own inactivity and to make themselves feel better about that by trying to make you feel worse.

I seriously doubt that the people making this prediction know that several studies comparing long-time runners to sedentary people have shown no difference in the rate at which people got arthritis. Also, studies comparing 55-and-older arthritis sufferers have found that over a five-year period, both the runners' and the nonrunners' arthritis got worse at the same rate. In other words, even in people who already had arthritis (which is often inherited), running didn't make it worse.

In fact, most experts agree that running can help against arthritis. First, weight-bearing exercise such as running strengthens bones and keeps joints better lubricated; "Use it or lose it" doesn't apply just to muscles. Second, you'll probably lose weight once you become a runner, and weighing less places less of a strain on your skeletal system than does forcing it to cart around an extra 30 pounds.

"Women are too fragile to run."

Supposedly well-meaning men have been throwing this myth around for centuries. It's usually just an excuse to perpetuate sexism. For example, when the Olympics were restarted in 1896, the International Olympic Committee wrote "that the Olympic Games must be reserved for the solemn and periodic exaltation of male athleticism."

Although women were fighting to get equal racing opportunities, they were being warned about the "dangers" of running from the medical community. In ancient times, Aristotle wrote that men have more teeth than women because it seemed logical to him; apparently, it never occurred to him to look in his wife's mouth and count. In the same way, even as recently as 20 years ago, women runners were told that they were risking sagging breasts, fallen ovaries, and infertility, even though no evidence exists to support these claims.

Footnotes

It wasn't until the 1928 Games that women were allowed to race even as far as 800 meters, which is just less than half a mile. A few ill-trained women collapsed at the end of these races, so all races of longer than 200 meters were banned from Olympic competition. (Isn't it interesting that when women collapse at the end of a race, they're thought to be frail, but when men do so, they're said to be so gutsy for having pushed themselves so hard?) The 800 meters wasn't put back on the program until 1960. There wasn't a women's Olympic marathon until 1984, a 10K until 1988, and a 5K until 1996!

Training affects women the same way that it does men—with more running, cardiovascular fitness improves, body fat decreases, and so on. Yes, on average, women will always be slower than men, owing to biological differences (some of which are related to childbirth) such as higher essential body fat stores. But stating that fact is different than saying that women are at risk from running.

Still think that women are too frail to run? Consider that it's in ultramarathons (races of 30 miles and longer) that women's performance comes closest to men's. Why is that? The leading theory can't be proved in a lab, but it sounds right to me: In these ultra-endurance events, where a big part of the battle is mental, women are simply tougher than men.

Footnotes

In 1994 and 1995, Ann Trason placed second overall at the Western States 100-miler, a California trail race.

The Least You Need to Know

➤ Among the leading reasons to run regularly are to lose weight, prevent disease, and have more energy and self-esteem.

➤ Running is the most convenient form of vigorous exercise.

➤ By one measure, there are more than 8 million regular runners in the United States.

➤ Runners come in all shapes, sizes, and ages.

➤ There's no real difference between running and jogging.

➤ Running doesn't cause arthritis.

Run for the Health of It

Most people start running for health reasons. They want to lose weight, have more energy, protect themselves against heart disease, or they just want to feel better. Any one of these reasons is powerful enough not only to start running, but also to stay motivated enough to keep at it.

The great thing about the health benefits of running is how they work together to reinforce each other. For example, running to lose weight also helps your heart and bones, and feeling better physically also improves your psychological health. This chapter details some of the main health benefits of running and points out how they work together to make your life better.

Lose the Fat

Everyone knows that it's bad to be overweight. Obese people (people who weigh at least 20 percent more than their ideal weight) are three times as likely as people of normal weight to develop high blood pressure and five times as likely to develop diabetes. Some doctors claim that obesity causes more than 300,000 early deaths a year in the United States. Look around the next time you're at a mall or an airport, where you can see a good cross-section of Americans, and you'll see that this problem is getting worse, not better, despite the fitness boom of the last 20 years. Nearly 60 million Americans are obese—almost one in four!

You don't have to be obese to have a reason to shed some pounds, however. By some measures, more than half of all Americans carry too much weight. Even though these people are not obese, they're still placing additional stress on their hearts, bones, and joints. Maybe you have an extra 10 pounds that seems to have tacked itself on to your middle sometime in the last few years. What you want to know is whether running can help you to trim down. The short answer is: Of course it can.

Weight for It

Running to lose weight is one of the single most popular reasons that people take up the sport, for good reason. Look around the next time you find yourself at a road race. See many overweight people finishing the race? That's not meant to imply that only runners who finish races lose weight. I just wanted to reinforce what most people know intuitively—regular runners are less likely to have problems with their weight than most people. That fact is important to remember if losing weight is one of your main motivations to start running. Why? Because although weight loss through running can be dramatic, it takes time.

Footnotes

Who knows what might be hiding under that extra layer of flab? Fifteen years ago, Peter Maher was a 210-pound smoker. Now, he's run a 2:11 marathon and has represented Canada in the Olympics.

Nearly all of our society is based on quick results and instant gratification. Need cash? There's an ATM around the corner. Article in the morning paper bother you? Fire off an e-mail to the editor. Dying to know the temperature in Outer Mongolia? Just turn on The Weather Channel. I'm all in favor of convenience. Unfortunately, though, the notion that everything can and should happen quickly has crept into areas of our lives where that's just not how things happen. Those areas include weight loss.

Although seemingly half the magazines in the world carry the line, "Lose 10 pounds before breakfast!" on their covers, that's just not how it works. If losing weight were that easy, then more than half of Americans wouldn't be overweight. Taking off your extra flab takes time and patience. After all, you didn't gain your spare tire overnight, so you shouldn't expect to lose it overnight.

Depressed yet? Don't be. As I said, most people know that regular runners are less likely to be overweight. I'll spend pretty much the rest of this book showing you various ways to become and remain a regular runner. Do that and some (if not all) of the extra weight that you may be carrying around will disappear.

The Math of Losing Weight

So how do you lose weight by running? A pound of body fat contains 3,500 *calories*. Covering a mile on foot, either by walking or running, burns approximately 100 calories. The exact number depends on your weight, the terrain you cover, your fitness, and other factors, but the difference is small enough that 100 calories per mile is an applicable figure for all people. At the most basic level, you lose one pound of body fat for every 35 miles you run.

I know what you're thinking: That's a lot of running just to lose one pound! Isn't there anything you can do to speed the process? Yes, there is. Let's look at the math more carefully. OK, so you burn 100 calories per mile. Say you're running 10 miles per week. You're creating a calorie deficit of 1,000 calories per week, so it will take you about three and a half weeks to burn a pound of body fat through running alone.

Track Talk
A *calorie* is a measurement of heat. Only foods containing calories can be burned for energy by your body. A pound is equal to 3,500 calories. Walking and running burn roughly 100 calories per mile.

But what if you make a few changes in your diet at the same time? What if you cut out that sugar-laden soda? There's 150 calories right there. What if you eat a banana instead of a chocolate chip cookie at lunch? There's another couple of hundred calories saved. Yes, you've probably tried dieting before, and it didn't work for you. That's not what I recommending here. Diets alone don't work. Continually denying yourself is too hard, and it's also not a healthy way to live. But combine a few small changes a day in your diet with exercise, and things are different.

Suppose you combine running 10 miles a week with making good "food trades" that save you 300 calories a day. Suddenly, you're at a calorie deficit of more than 3,000 per week, or nearly enough to lose one pound a week. That's a safe level of weight loss. If you lose four to five pounds per month, it starts adding up.

Making running, not dieting, the main focus of your weight-loss program works in part because you're doing something positive (running) to shed the pounds rather than not

Training Tip
Don't weigh yourself more than once a week. Your weight varies from day to day because of water retention and other factors, so daily weighings can be misleading and frustrating. Try to weigh yourself under similar conditions each week, such as naked on Monday mornings.

doing something fun (eating). If you follow my advice in this book, then you'll come to enjoy your running, and the lost weight will be just one of the many things that you value it for.

In addition, exercise, not diet, is the way to go because after you work out, your metabolism remains elevated for hours. One study found that after an easy hour run, subjects were still burning calories at an accelerated rate more than seven hours later! Even after a 30-minute run, their metabolism was revved up for two hours after finishing. So by running, you're burning extra calories even when you're at rest. That doesn't happen with dieting. In fact, the opposite does. Also, every bit of muscle that you gain with your running helps you to lose weight. Muscles burn more calories at rest than fat does.

Just Run

You may have heard about special "fat-burning" workouts that draw exclusively from your fat stores and speed your weight loss. Runners are often told that running at a lower intensity will burn more fat than running faster. That's true, but incomplete and misleading.

Here's the deal: When you're sitting in a chair, you're burning almost nothing but fat. As your activity level increases, your muscles start to burn *glycogen*, which is how your body stores most of the carbohydrates that you eat. Glycogen is your muscles' preferred fuel source for exercise. The harder you work out toward a maximal effort, the percentage of the calories burned from glycogen increases, and the percentage that comes from fat decreases. When you're sprinting all out, you're burning no fat at all.

Track Talk
Glycogen is your body's main source of fuel during aerobic exercise. It's stored in your muscles and liver, and then burned when you work out. With training, you increase your body's capacity to store glycogen, but even well-trained runners can usually store only enough for 20 or so miles of running.

Based on that information, some people will say to work out at a very easy pace to burn more fat. Technically, that's true. But as the previous example shows, if you want to do nothing but burn fat, sit down. You'll be burning almost nothing else!

What matters is not where the calories come from that you burn, but how many you burn. As I said, whether you walk or run, you burn about 100 calories per mile. So if you walk three miles, you'll burn 300 calories, and more of those calories will come from your fat stores than if you run three miles. But think about the time involved. Walking three miles is going to take close to an hour for most people. In the same amount of time, you could probably run twice as far. The result? You'll have burned twice as many calories, and that's what matters in taking and keeping the pounds off.

That's why running is so great for losing weight. In just half an hour, you can burn as many calories as you would doing many other exercises for an hour or more. Running's convenience and the short time each day that you need to allot for it mean that it's easy to do regularly, meaning that you're more likely to burn more calories more often.

Composition Exercise

How do you know if you need to lose weight? This question is tricky, with everyone's situation being different. But ask yourself this: Were you a healthy, active person in your early 20s? If so, what did you weigh then? Do you weigh more now? You shouldn't. By your early 20s, you're pretty much done growing (at least vertically!). Unless you've spent most days in the gym since then lifting weights, it's probably not an extra 20 pounds of muscle you've gained.

Overall, it's better to focus on your *body composition* than exclusively on your weight. Your body composition is what percentage of your weight is lean body mass (muscles, bones, and everything else that isn't fat) and what percentage is fat (both the fat stored in and around organs of your body and what you can see or feel beneath your skin). Concentrating on body composition recognizes that you can be very fit, but still be "overweight" by common standards.

Measurements of body composition get people to realize that you can be at what the weight charts would tell you is a "desirable" weight, but still not be fit, or even healthy. Think about how many people keep smoking because they don't want to gain 10 pounds. You can starve yourself and be at a "desirable" weight, but be doing major damage to your body. It's how your body is constructed, not just how many pounds it weighs, that's important.

A good way to determine whether you have a decent body composition is by calculating your body mass index. This involves some math, so get out the calculator and follow these steps:

Training Tip
Are you carrying too much fat? Try this quick test: While standing with erect posture, grab a section of flesh between your thumb and fingers, about one to two inches to the side of your navel. If the fold of skin is less than an inch thick, then you probably don't need to worry about excess body fat.

Track Talk
Your *body composition* is a measure of how much fat you're carrying compared to lean tissue. Generally, the lower your level of body fat, the less you are at risk for disease, the better you feel moving around, and the better you look!

1. Determine your weight in kilograms by multiplying your weight in pounds by 0.454.

2. Determine your height in meters by multiplying your height in inches by 0.0254.

3. Square your height in meters (multiply it by itself).

4. Divide your weight in kilograms by the square of your height in meters.

The result is your body mass index. For example, if you are 5'10" and weigh 150 pounds, you would multiply 150 by 0.454, for a weight in kilograms of 68.1. Your height in inches is 70; multiply that by 0.0254 for a height in meters of 1.778. Square that number to get 3.16. Finally, divide 68.1 (weight in kilograms) by 3.16 (square of height in meters) to get a body mass index of 21.5. Desirable body mass index ranges are 19 to 25 for both men and women. If your index is above 25, you probably are carrying too much fat.

Of course, you may not need to do this test. For many people, a look in the mirror while naked does the trick. Is the waist in your jeans a few inches more than when you were in your early 20s? Has your shirt or dress size increased? As I said, unless you've been training with Arnold Schwarzenegger, your clothes probably fit differently because of gaining fat, not muscle. Running can help you to lose the extra fat.

Disease Flees

Many runners are perfectly content with their weight, but keep running for other health reasons. When you run regularly, your aerobic capacity increases. The exercise scientists refer to this capacity as maximal oxygen uptake, or VO₂ *max*. Whatever you call it, it refers to your body's plumbing for aerobic exercise. Runners with a high VO₂ max have a plumbing system that allows them to pump large amounts of oxygen-rich blood to working muscles. With training, you can maximize the size of your pump and the quantity of blood that it transports.

Track Talk
The scientific term for your aerobic capacity is maximal oxygen uptake, or VO₂ *max*. It's a measure of how much oxygen your body can deliver to working muscles. Most people's maximal oxygen uptake increases by 20 to 30 percent in the first year of running.

With six months to a year of training, previously sedentary people can expect to increase their aerobic capacity by 20 percent to 30 percent. That's a large part of why you're able to run substantially farther and faster after a few months of regular running than before you started. For racers, working to improve their VO₂ max is one of the most important parts of their training. For our purposes here, though, what's significant is that as your aerobic capacity increases, your risk for some of the most common debilitating diseases of modern society decreases.

Handling Heart Disease

The American Heart Association (AHA) lists four major risk factors for developing coronary artery disease: smoking, high blood pressure, high blood cholesterol levels, and lack of regular exercise. In other words, even if you don't smoke and have acceptable blood pressure and cholesterol levels, you're still at an increased risk for heart disease if you're sedentary.

Footnotes

The AHA used to count lack of exercise as a contributing, not a major factor. But in 1992 they revised their standards because an increasing number of studies showed that even when similar in every other way, a sedentary person is almost twice as likely to have heart disease than a regular exerciser.

The reason why running and other aerobic exercise dramatically reduce your risk for heart disease isn't difficult to discern. As your aerobic capacity increases, your heart becomes more efficient and powerful. By stressing it for a short time at least a few times a week, you lessen the stress on it all the rest of the time.

Running also works to lower your other risk factors. Running helps to prevent or delay the development of high blood pressure, and it helps to control it in people who have a genetic predisposition to the condition. Running also helps to lower your overall blood cholesterol level, and running is one of the greatest ways to quit smoking.

In other words, if you start running, you not only remove one of the major risks for developing heart disease (being sedentary), but you also go a long way toward eliminating the others. To top it all off, running can also help with what the AHA identifies as contributing factors toward heart disease, including obesity, stress, and diabetes. No wonder that one famous study of Harvard alumni, led by Ralph Paffenbarger, Ph.D., found that those who burned at least 2,000 calories a week in vigorous exercise (about 20 miles a week) were 64 percent less likely to suffer a heart attack than their sedentary contemporaries.

Better Bones

Studies show a direct link between regular weight-bearing exercise, such as running, and bone thickness. The stronger a bone, the more stress it can handle before it breaks. This health benefit is especially important for women runners. Everyone starts losing bone mineral density after the age of 30. When women are past menopause, their estrogen levels drop, and their bones lose even more density. But running, along with a diet rich in calcium, can halt this loss. The upshot is that runners are less likely to suffer from osteoporosis, a disease in which bones become brittle and break easily.

Footnotes

The strongest link between aerobic exercise and lower cancer risk is in colon cancer. Studies have found that regular exercisers have about half the incidence of colon cancer as sedentary people do. There's also increasing evidence to suggest a lower risk of breast cancer among active women.

Breathe Easy

A key component of increased aerobic capacity is better lung function. Just as your heart becomes stronger with regular running, so do your lungs. They're able to sustain a higher work load for a longer period of time. As your lungs become more efficient, you can take in more oxygen with each breath. That's one of the reasons why you don't breathe as hard climbing stairs when you're fit—your lungs are better able to get oxygen to working muscles.

In terms of medical conditions, this better lung function means that people who have asthma not only can run, but should do some form of regular exercise. After all, when you improve your body's capacity to take in and use oxygen, then what it considers stressful occurs at a much higher level of exertion. So an activity that previously might have triggered an asthma attack doesn't as you become fitter. Also, because your breathing becomes smoother as you get fit, there's less chance that your airways will become irritated.

Footnotes

Asthmatics can be athletes, too. Of the 597 members of the 1984 U.S. Olympic team, more than 10 percent had asthma.

The other big breathing-related benefit of running is one that I've mentioned before: It can help you to stop smoking. Remember what I said about how most people know that regular runners don't have as many weight problems as sedentary people? Well, the same is true with respect to running and smoking. You just don't see the two mix after awhile.

I know from my experience that when I started running again, smoking became increasingly less attractive. Yes, I still smoked when I started running again in the early '70s.

Nicotine is addictive, after all. But I knew that if I stuck with the running, my body would eventually get so fed up with me continuing to poison it that I would eventually be able to kick my habit. Take my word on it: As your system becomes cleaner and more efficient, it becomes more sensitive to things that damage it. Few things are more damaging to it than cigarettes.

Head Games

You've probably heard about "the runner's high." The definitions are never all that precise, but it's supposed to be some sort of transcendent state that you enter into after running for half an hour or so. Many beginning runners have been told about the runner's high and figure that they must be doing things wrong, because they've certainly never felt like Timothy Leary on a run.

I'm here to tell you that the runner's high is an overblown concept. There's no such thing as a quantifiable, yes-or-no transcendent state that X amount of running induces, any more than listening to 3.4 of your favorite songs causes a definitive change in your mental condition. So don't belittle or doubt yourself because you're not achieving the runner's high—in one sense, there's no such thing to achieve.

But like music, running does have a dramatic effect on your mood. Let me be the first to tell you that if you don't finish most of your runs feeling calmer, more content, relaxed, and less tense and angst-ridden, then you're doing something wrong. If you want to call that a runner's high, I'm not going to argue. Short-term stress relief is one of the main things that gets busy runners out the door. Studies have found that people score much lower on tests of anxiety immediately after finishing a run, compared to how they scored before their run. As one knowledgeable running doctor has noted, even as little as 15 minutes of moderate walking reduces muscular tension more than a standard dose of a tranquilizer.

Over the long haul, those psychological benefits accrue. Indeed, aerobic exercise, such as running, is a common prescription for mild depression. Less dramatically, but just as important, runners consistently rate higher than average on these important personality characteristics:

➤ Emotional stability

➤ Optimism

➤ Self-sufficiency

➤ Self-esteem

Compared to sedentary people, runners have also been found to have an increased ability to concentrate and above average organizational and problem solving skills. They also report feeling content and mentally vigorous more often than do nonexercisers. In other words, running clears your brain along with your arteries.

Footnotes

The International Society of Sport Psychology says the following in a position statement, "Physical Activity and Psychological Benefits": "Individual psychological benefits of physical activity include positive changes in self-perception and well-being, improvement in self-confidence and awareness, positive changes in mood, relief of tension, relief of feelings such as depression and anxiety, influence on premenstrual tension, increased mental well-being, increased alertness and clear thinking, increased energy and ability to cope with daily activity, increased enjoyment of exercise and social contacts, and development of positive coping strategies."

Why does running put you in a better mood? The answer is endorphins. These chemicals, which act like morphine, are released by your brain when you're under stress. Studies have found that the level of endorphins circulating in your system can be more than twice as high after a run compared to when you're at rest.

Training Tip

When you're under a lot of stress, be more diligent than usual about making time to run. Those endorphins that flood your body will go a long way toward keeping you calm enough to work through your problems.

In the long term, there's less of a chemical explanation for why running is so good for you psychologically. Nonetheless, the reasons seem pretty clear to me. For starters, as you become more fit, you're going to have a better self-image. You'll feel better about how you look and about your health. By being less absorbed with self-loathing, you can turn your attention toward having a brighter outlook toward the world.

In addition, setting and achieving goals on a regular basis is tremendously satisfying. After almost every run, you'll have a feeling of accomplishment—you overcame inertia, got out the door, and did something good for yourself. Being able to remind yourself that you wanted to work out four times last week and did so can bring a boost when events seem to be directing you, rather than you directing them.

Adding Life to Your Years

If you've been paying attention during this chapter, you've probably already concluded what I'm about to say: One of the greatest health benefits of running is how all of the many wonderful things it does for your body and mind work together. You feel more at home in your body, you don't get as tired doing normal activities, you feel better about yourself, you're more regularly in a better mood—these aren't the kinds of things that can necessarily be quantified in medical terms, but I defy anyone to tell me that they don't go a long way toward improving your health.

Some people refer to this snowball effect of running's benefits as putting more life in your years. When you're a runner, you're more able to use your body as you want to, which makes you feel more alive. Life might not be any easier, but living it sure is. Any long-time runner will tell you that his or her quality of life is significantly higher since becoming a runner. That's what vitality is all about.

So running adds life to your years. But does running add years to your life? The answer is yes. As a Surgeon General's report in 1996 put it, "higher levels of regular physical activity are associated with lower mortality rates for both older and younger adults." In other words, when you compare runners and other exercisers to sedentary people, the active ones are more likely to outlive the couch potatoes.

Remember that study of Harvard grads that I mentioned when talking about heart disease? In that section, I explained that burning at least 2,000 calories a week in vigorous activity, which is the rough equivalent of running 20 miles a week, significantly lowers your risk for having heart disease. The same study found that the 20 miles per week threshold also coincides with longer lives. Participants in the study who maintained that level of activity from age 35 onward outlived the less active subjects by two and a half years.

And it's never too late: Even those who waited until after the age of 50 to start that seemingly magic 2,000 calories a week level of exercise gained an extra one to two years. Put all of these benefits together, and you not only have extra years of life, but you also feel great during more years of that life. Can you believe that some people *don't* run?

The Least You Need to Know

> ➤ Running is a better way to lose weight and keep it off than dieting.
> ➤ You burn the equivalent of one pound of body fat for every 35 miles you run.
> ➤ Running can cut your risk of heart disease in half.
> ➤ Runners have stronger bones and lungs than sedentary people.
> ➤ Runners have more self-esteem, self-confidence, and mental alertness than sedentary people.
> ➤ Running at least 20 miles a week can increase your life span by more than two years.

Taking Your First Steps

In This Chapter

➤ What to do before you start running

➤ How to get started

➤ How to increase your endurance

➤ Running at the right pace

➤ Running with good form

Who said that the journey of a lifetime begins with a single step? Whoever it was understood what it's like to be a new runner. After all, even the most experienced marathoners out there at one point took their first running step. I certainly remember how momentous my first ones seemed when I started running in the early '70s.

So don't worry; we were all beginners once. Try not to let fear of the unknown deter you from running. Follow what I say in this chapter, and you'll be able to progress safely and satisfactorily from your current state of activity to being a regular runner.

Doctor's Orders?

I'm not a doctor; I don't even play one on TV. So I'm not going to claim to be qualified to dole out medical advice. Unfortunately, when it comes to running, a lot of doctors aren't experts, either. It's become almost reflexive to say that anyone thinking about starting a running program should get medical clearance first. Well, I'm going to be a bit different and not take cover under that blanket statement.

Why? A few reasons, none of which are meant to put down the medical profession. But consider this statistic: Even after the last 25 years of the fitness boom, less than 30 percent of doctors advise their patients about exercise and nutrition. Doctors are trained to fight disease, not prescribe health. I've had more than one doctor ask me if I'm amazed that my knees haven't given out yet.

There's a kind of philosophical basis to my argument. To me, it seems that saying that everyone has to get medical clearance before starting to run implies that running is some dangerous activity, not one of the best things you can do to take control of your health. You're preparing to go outside and use your body as it's meant to be used, not preparing to be sent to battle.

Why do so many people say that you should run only with a note from your doctor? In part, the reason is because running is portrayed so inaccurately in the general media. Every year, about 30,000 people run the New York City Marathon. Every few years, one of those runners has a heart attack during the race. Sadly, sometimes the runner dies. This tragedy is what gets play in the papers.

But did you know that at the University of Michigan's home football games, the medical teams expect to treat two heart attack patients per game from the stands? That's what the law of averages would tell you is going to happen when you have 100,000 people together in one place. Do you then see the media warning about the risks of watching football games?

Rules of the Road
Be honest with yourself when you're assessing whether you should see a doctor before starting to run. Running doesn't cause heart problems, but if you have an underlying one, it can aggravate it.

If I sound a little sensitive here, it's partly because of the attention the media gave when Jim Fixx died of a heart attack while running in 1984. Because Fixx was the author of the best-selling *The Complete Book of Running*, he was a spokesperson for the sport. I know a lot of people who subsequently quit running, because they figured that if running killed Jim Fixx, who wasn't at risk?

I knew Jim Fixx. What was not reported was that heart disease ran in his family and that even with dying at age 52, Fixx had already outlived his father by nine years. More important—and here I might win back some of the doctors I've just angered—is that Fixx thought that his marathon running made him immune and so ignored his medical history. He had been a heavy smoker before he started running, and his cholesterol levels were way above normal. He also ignored chest pains that he sometimes got while running, as well as pleas from Kenneth Cooper, M.D.,(sometimes called the father of aerobics) to get regular check-ups.

Am I contradicting myself here? Not at all. Everyone should know their medical history, as well as that of their family. I'm assuming that you get regular physicals, know your blood pressure and cholesterol level, and so on. If you don't, and if starting a running program inspires you to see a doctor, then by all means go. I just worry sometimes that getting a doctor's "permission" to run keeps a lot of people from ever starting.

So besides those who don't know their basic health information, who should see a doctor before starting a running program? The National Heart, Lung, and Blood Institute has issued the following guidelines, and they seem reasonable to me. If one of these statements applies to you, discuss your desire to start a running program with a doctor, preferably one who is used to treating active patients.

➤ You're over the age of 60 and aren't used to regular exercise.

➤ You have family members who have had coronary artery disease before the age of 55.

➤ You frequently have pain or feel pressure in the left or mid chest area, the left side of your neck, the left shoulder, or left arm during or immediately after exercise.

➤ You often feel faint, dizzy, or unaccountably out of breath after mild exertion.

➤ You have high blood pressure that isn't under control.

➤ You've had heart trouble, a heart murmur, or a heart attack.

➤ You have arthritis.

➤ You have a medical condition that might need special attention once you start exercising, such as diabetes.

If none of these statements applies to you, you can proceed to learning how to get going.

From 0 to 30 Minutes in a Month

There's no universally applicable program for starting a running program. As I stress again and again in this book, regardless of whether I'm talking about how to build endurance or why to run or even what shoes to wear, running is an individual sport. As the old saying goes, every runner is an experiment of one. What works for one runner might be a disaster for another. All runners are going to progress at different rates.

Still, there are a few basic guidelines that all runners should follow. In telling you how to get going, I'll give these guidelines to you. You might find what I recommend either too easy or too hard. If either of these conditions is the case, that's fine. The guiding principle in your running should always be to stay in tune with what you feel comfortable with.

Walk, Don't Run

This advice might sound strange, but the best way to start a running program for a lot of people is to walk. That's especially the case if you haven't been active for the last few years or are overweight. I know, you bought a book on running. You want to run! But when it comes to starting a regular running routine, slow and steady is always going to win the race.

Now, I'm not going to lie to you: When you're new to running, especially if you've been sedentary, running is going to hurt for awhile. Later I'll explain how it should and shouldn't hurt, but I wanted to get that out on the table from the get-go. You're asking your body to do something that it's not accustomed to. Initially, your body is going to protest. You're going to be a little sore and, at first, a little more tired.

Footnotes

Don't try this at home: When Patti Catalano, who eventually held the American record in the marathon, decided to start a running program, her first run was seven miles. She could barely walk, much less run, for more than a week afterwards.

Your body is going to protest really loudly if you overload it too much right off the bat. If you try to do too much too soon, the soreness and fatigue are going to be so great that you're going to have stop for several days at a time. When you start again, you'll be starting from scratch. Then you might feel as if you're behind schedule and might overdo it that much more. Bad idea!

Training Tip
Start all of your workouts at a little slower pace than you think you need to. This slower pace gives your muscles and your heart and breathing rates a chance to warm up and increase gradually. You'll feel better if you ease into your workouts.

A better idea is acknowledging that you're going to be sore and a little fatigued at first and doing what you can to minimize those inevitabilities. For a lot of people, that's going to mean walking at first, then gradually introducing some bouts of easy running, and then gradually increasing the length of those bouts.

The biggest battle that all runners face is sticking with it. Even long-time runners can find it tough to find a routine that works for them. What's most important at first is getting in the habit of exercising regularly. Erring on the side of caution when you start is going to help you to feel good enough to stick with it. As you become fitter, you'll already have your exercise routine down and can progress toward more running. So get out the door and start walking. When doing so is comfortable for you, report back, and I'll get going on making you a runner.

When to Run, When to Rest

What's a good routine to get into? I recommend that beginners shoot for half an hour, four days a week. Mind you, I don't mean half an hour of running four times a week right off the bat. In the schedule at the end of this section, I'll show you how to gradually build to being able to run 30 minutes at a time.

What I'm assuming in this chart is that at the start of the first week, you can handle walking at a brisk pace for half an hour at a time, four times a week. If you can't, then don't start the running portions of the schedule yet. Keep walking until you have that basic level of fitness that will allow you to walk for half an hour, four times a week.

If you've been doing a little running already, it's OK to jump into the chart at the level you're at. For example, if you know that you can run a mile, then it's OK to enter the schedule at the point where I have you running for 10 minutes straight at a stretch. But if you're going to do that, you have to promise to be honest with yourself. There's a big difference between knowing that you can run a mile because you did it once a few weeks ago and doing so four times in a week. If you don't run regularly, be conservative and enter the schedule at about half the level that you know you can handle in one run. So if you know that you can run a mile but haven't been doing so a few times a week, start where the schedule has you running for five minutes at a time.

> **Training Tip**
> Getting fit is hard enough on its own. Make doing so easier by doing your early walking and running on terrain as flat as you can find.

The reason behind this advice is an important principle that applies to all runners, from the most out-of-shape beginner to the fastest runners in the world. It's the *progression principle*. What it says is that the way to improve your fitness is gradually, in small, consistent steps, rather than in great leaps.

> **Track Talk**
> The *progression principle* says that individual gains in fitness are small, but accumulate with consistency. That's why you can't go from being inactive to running a marathon; you have to gradually increase your endurance.

Consistency is the single most important factor in determining whether you'll improve as a runner. Becoming a runner is like saving for retirement. The best way is to start small, but be consistent, and then build on your earlier progress. As you accumulate money for retirement or improve your fitness level, you can see the progress that you're making and will be motivated to keep at it. No one day is a great transformative event, where you suddenly have a lot more money or can suddenly run three times farther than usual. You chip away at it, and what once seemed impossible—setting aside $10,000, or running for 15 minutes without stopping—becomes just another signpost on the way to your next goal.

In retirement savings, progress happens because of interest. In running, progress happens because of how your body works. You give it this new task of running just a bit. Your body is a little shocked and thinks, "Hmm, I haven't really experienced that before. This crazy person just might ask me to do that again. I had better be ready." So it prepares itself in order to be just a little more capable of handling what you did to it recently.

Gain Through Pain

You're sore when you start working out regularly because you've done microscopic damage to your muscles, and they're irritated. But give them the chance to recover from that short-term damage, and they'll rebuild themselves to be a little bit stronger and better able to work at the level that they think you're going to ask them to again. The same goes for other body parts, such as your heart and lungs.

When you make another little progression in effort, the same thing happens again. This process is never too great a stress, but a stress nonetheless. After a few rounds of this, your body catches on that this is going to become a regular process. The result is that it fortifies itself, and you become fitter.

Now, if you've been paying attention during this extended narrative, you'll have noted a crucial fact: The important gains in fitness come not while you're running, but after you run. That's an example of the *stress/recovery principle*. To put this principle into practice, you stress your body, which tears it down a little. Then you give your body a chance to recover, and while recovering, you body rebuilds itself to be just a little more capable of handling the next bout of similar stress.

Track Talk
The *stress/ recovery principle* says that you become fitter by subjecting your body to a stress, and then allowing recovery time before you stress it again. During the recovery time, the body rebuilds itself to be better able to handle that stress. In the case of running, this principle means that your heart, lungs, and muscles become stronger between running sessions.

In other words, providing adequate recovery is the key to progressing. That's why you can't hurry your way from being sedentary to fit. You have to allow your body time between workouts to become stronger. If you don't allow time, you're going to plateau. That's why I think you should start with four days a week—you're going often enough to make progress, but not so much that you can't recover between workouts.

But don't some runners run every day? What about their need for recovery time? One of the benefits of becoming fit is that your recovery time between workouts shortens dramatically. Most top runners train twice a day. Their bodies have become so accustomed to the stress/recovery process that they can do two runs within the space of eight hours and feel fine on both. But even they're not immune to the same principles that beginners are. When they do more than they're used to and don't allow enough time between hard efforts, they get sore and tired, just like you.

A Beginner's Schedule

A word about the following schedule: I don't know what your usual week is like, so it would be silly for me to say that you have to start your workout week on Sunday, then go again on Tuesday, Wednesday, and Saturday. When you go is going to depend on when the workout meshes best with the rest of your life. So in the schedule, I've marked workouts as the first one of the week rather than noting on which days to do them. What's important is following the progression and planning your workouts so that you have that crucial recovery time between workouts. In other words, try not to do the four workouts for a week on four consecutive days.

And now, at last, a schedule of how to progress from 0 to 30 minutes of running in a month. Remember, before starting workout 1 of week 1, you should already be able to walk for 30 minutes, four times a week. If you can't do a given workout, don't worry. Stay with that one until you can and move on to the next one only after you've mastered the prior one.

Before—and especially after—your workout, it's a good idea to do some gentle stretching. See Chapter 10 for more details.

Week 1

Workout 1: Walk 10 minutes. Then, for the next 10 minutes, alternate running for 1 minute with walking for 1 minute. Walk 10 minutes.

Workout 2: Walk 10 minutes. Then, for the next 15 minutes, alternate running for 1 minute with walking for 1 minute. Walk 5 minutes.

Workout 3: Walk 10 minutes. Then, for the next 15 minutes, alternate running for 2 minutes with walking for 1 minute. Walk 5 minutes.

Workout 4: Walk 5 minutes. Then, for 21 minutes, alternate running for 2 minutes with walking for 1 minute. Walk 4 minutes.

Week 2

Workout 1: Walk 5 minutes. Then, for the next 20 minutes, alternate running for 3 minutes with walking for 1 minute. Walk 5 minutes.

Workout 2: Walk 5 minutes. Then, for the next 21 minutes, alternate running for 5 minutes with walking for 2 minutes. Walk 4 minutes.

Workout 3: Walk 4 minutes. Then, for the next 24 minutes, alternate running for 5 minutes with walking for 1 minute. Walk 2 minutes.

Workout 4: Walk 5 minutes. Then, for the next 22 minutes, alternate running for 8 minutes with walking for 3 minutes. Walk 3 minutes.

Week 3

Workout 1: Walk 5 minutes. Run 10 minutes. Walk 5 minutes. Run 5 minutes. Walk 5 minutes.

Workout 2: Walk 5 minutes. Run 12 minutes. Walk 3 minutes. Run 5 minutes. Walk 5 minutes.

Workout 3: Walk 10 minutes. Run 15 minutes. Walk 5 minutes.

Workout 4: Walk 6 minutes. Run 18 minutes. Walk 6 minutes.

Week 4

Workout 1: Walk 5 minutes. Run 20 minutes. Walk 5 minutes.

Workout 2: Walk 5 minutes. Run 22 minutes. Walk 3 minutes.

Workout 3: Walk 3 minutes. Run 25 minutes. Walk 2 minutes.

Workout 4: Run 30 minutes.

Running on at the Mouth: The Talk Test

Most people think that running means being constantly out of breath. Most beginners contribute to this misconception because, believe it or not, they run too fast. They think that running is always supposed to be hard work, so the more difficult it feels, the more correctly they're doing it, and the more they're benefiting; but that's not the case.

Most runners should run at a relaxed, moderate pace just this side of being out of breath for most of their running sessions. That's certainly always been the case for me, even when I was training to be the best in the world. At this pace, you train, but don't strain. You're providing that slight stress to your body that's going to prompt it to get stronger, but you're running within yourself rather than going all out.

How do you know what this pace is? In scientific terms, it corresponds to getting your heart rate up to about 70 percent of its maximum. In Chapter 9, I'll tell you more about the benefits of monitoring your training based on tracking your heart rate.

Of course, most runners, especially most beginners, don't know what these figures are to begin with, much less use them for training. But that's not a problem. You don't need a battery of tests and a heart rate monitor to find your optimal training pace; you don't even need to check how fast per mile you're running. All you need to do is strike up a conversation. When you can do so while running, but still feel as though you're putting in a solid effort, you're training at the right pace. This is known as passing the *talk test*.

Track Talk
The *talk test* is a way to know whether you're running at the proper pace to boost your endurance. You should be able to carry on a conversation while you run. If you can only say one or two words at a time, you're running too fast for a beginner.

Passing the talk test means that you should be able to speak in complete sentences while you're running at a moderate training level. If you can only offer one-word grunts in response to another runner's questions, then you're going too fast for how hard you should be running during the first few months of your running program. As I said, this is the level of effort that I maintain on most of my runs. (The exceptions are when I've planned to do some running at race pace or faster to prepare for competition.)

Footnotes

When I used to race marathons, I would use a version of the talk test to evaluate my competition. If runners were still with me past the 15-mile mark, and I couldn't tell how tired they were by their breathing or form, I would ask them questions that required more than a word or two to answer. If they responded in complete sentences, I knew I had a race to the finish on my hands.

The next time you see a group of experienced runners, watch closely. I bet you that you're more than likely to see them carrying on a conversation, even at what might appear to be a startlingly quick pace. You should follow their example. On the other hand, if you can reel off a soliloquy from *Hamlet* without breaking stride, you might want to pick it up a bit.

Going too fast might seem like a good way to get past a more moderate progression, but you can't trick your body into getting fitter than it's ready to. When you run too fast, you're not going to be able to extend your distance as easily; when you're starting out, it's how far you can run, not how fast, that's more important in building your endurance. Also, when you run too hard all the time, you're more likely to get injured, and you're less likely to enjoy your running and want to stick with it.

Of course, a lot of beginners don't always have someone to run with, so it's tough to know if they can pass the talk test. After all, you're probably self-conscious enough as it is when you start a running program; you don't need to have your neighbors see you trotting down the street carrying on a conversation with yourself to add to things. An alternative to the talk test is to check to see whether you can hum a familiar tune to yourself for a line or two at a time.

Another good way to gauge your effort is by judging it against a scale called rating of perceived effort. Research has shown that once runners learn the scale, they can accurately say where they are on it. Here's one version of the scale:

Rating	Perception of effort
0	Nothing at all
0.5	Very, very weak (just noticeable)

Rating	Perception of effort
1	Very weak
2	Weak
3	Moderate
4	Somewhat strong
5	Strong
6	Strong
7	Very strong
8	Very strong
9	Very strong
10	Very, very strong (almost maximal)
>10	Maximal

When you're gradually building your endurance, you should be in the 3 to 4 range. That's a similar level of effort to being able to pass the talk test.

A Stitch in Time

A problem that many beginning runners encounter is side stitches. If you've ever had one, you know what I'm talking about; it's a sharp, sudden pain just below your rib cage that can double you over and make continuing to run a chore.

There are a lot of theories about what causes side stitches. Many people think they're caused by your diaphragm muscles cramping, either because those muscles, which help with breathing, aren't used to working hard or because someone has started a run too quickly. This theory sounds right to me because beginners get stitches more often than do long-time runners. Veterans' muscles are obviously more accustomed to regular exertion, and experienced runners know to ease into their runs. In contrast, as I said previously, beginners often start their runs too quickly.

Sharp pains in your stomach might also be from something as simple as eating too soon before a run. This is another reason that beginners might experience stitches more than veterans because new runners often haven't learned how long they need to wait to eat after running or what foods don't mix well with their running.

Footnotes

Beginners aren't the only ones who are occasionally plagued by side stitches. Todd Williams, who is a two-time Olympian in the 10K, got such a bad side stitch in a 15K in March 1997 that he had to drop out of the race while leading.

The good news is that side stitches aren't a serious sort of problem, unlike if your foot starts throbbing a mile into most runs. If you get a side stitch, stop and walk. Concentrate on taking deep breaths. Exhale forcibly with your lips pursed. The stitch will usually go away in a minute or two. Then review how long ago you ate before your run and what you ate. Also, assess whether you began your run at an easy pace and increased your speed gradually only after you felt warmed up.

Running the Right Way

People worry too much about running form. Some books get so detailed in telling you how to run that you'd almost have to carry them with you when you run to make sure you're getting it right. How your feet should land, where they should land, how long your stride should be, what to do with your hands, how to hold your arms—I'd trip after a few hundred yards if I spent my runs thinking about this stuff. I'm not saying that good running form isn't important or that you can't or shouldn't try to improve yours. But running isn't a technique sport like golf. It's a lot easier to tell people how to have as sweet a stroke as Tiger Woods' than it is to say that all runners should run in one precise way.

We all run like we do for a reason, namely, according to how our bodies are put together. Look around, and you'll notice that no two bodies are put together the same. Some people's legs are bowed. Some people's feet are flatter than others. Some people have wider hips than others, or leg muscles that are stronger, or back muscles that are weaker. All of these factors determine what kind of running form you have.

Remember, each runner is an experiment of one. One of my legs is longer than the other. As a result, I land on the extreme outside edge of my left forefoot, and my right arm often swings across my body. This is not textbook form, but it's what works for me and what feels comfortable.

That last point is crucial. The best running form for you is the one that you feel most comfortable with. As you become fitter, your running form is going to become more natural to you, and you'll think about it less. Remember when you started driving a car? You were so concerned with how you were holding the wheel, the position of your feet, and so forth that you could barely pay attention to the road. Now, driving is second nature to you. Same thing for long-time runners. They just get out there and run and don't really think about how they're doing it all that much.

That's not to say that you should ignore your running form. Some basic points can help make running feel smoother and make you less susceptible to injury. Here are the most important ones:

➤ Upright posture, with your head, shoulders, torso, and pelvis aligned and your head held up and looking ahead, not down

➤ Arms carried low, with your shoulders relaxed

➤ Hands relaxed, cupped loosely, and passing your body at about waist level

➤ Arms moving in sync with your legs, driving forward, rather than from side to side

➤ Feet landing gently under your center of gravity

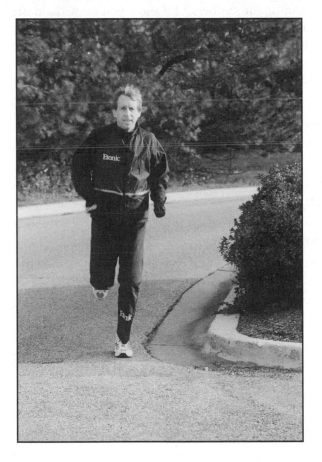

Notice how Bill's posture is upright and aligned, his arms are low and relaxed, and his left foot is landing under his center of gravity.

Training Tip
Don't try to change your form all at once or overnight. Pick an element that you want to work on. On some runs, think about how to improve that element, and concentrate on running slightly differently for 5 minutes at a time. For example, if your shoulders are usually hunched forward, try pulling them back and see how that feels while running.

And that's just for starters. I told you it was a lot to think about.

Is it worth it to try to improve your form? It can be if running doesn't feel comfortable once you attain a basic level of fitness. If you notice that you're often straining one body part, or that a certain body part, such as your shoulders, tires as you run, then it can be worth it to try to make a few adjustments.

But again, don't make too much out of comparing your form to others. As you become fitter, your form is going to get better because the muscles throughout your body that support you when you run are going to get more used to their new task. Also, in Chapter 11, "Pumped Up: Strength Training for Runners," I'll show you some basic strengthening exercises that can go a long way toward helping you run with better form.

The Least You Need to Know

➤ The best way to start a running program is by mixing walking and running and increasing the running portion as you become fitter.

➤ Prepare for the main part of your workout with a warm-up of gentle stretching and walking.

➤ After the main part of your run, ease the transition to a normal heart rate with walking and then more stretching.

➤ In the first few months of a running program, you should always go slow enough to be able to maintain a conversation.

➤ Side stitches are common for beginning runners and are usually caused by going too quickly.

➤ Instead of copying how others do it, run with the form that feels most comfortable for you.

Chapter 4

Strutting Your Stuff: Where to Run

In This Chapter

➤ Safety rules for running

➤ Finding good places to run

➤ The best surfaces for running

➤ Running while traveling

When you decide to start golfing, it's pretty obvious where to go to practice your new sport. Same thing with tennis, swimming, and a lot of other activities. Your venues are usually few and far between.

But when you become a runner, the world is your oyster. One of the great things about running, and one of the reasons that so many people can stick with it, is its convenience. You can run almost anywhere: streets, tracks, parks, trails, and so on. I even ran once on an airport runway in Venezuela, but that's something I'd rather not get into right now. My point is that with running, your options are almost infinite. Still, some surfaces are better than others. This chapter examines the advantages and disadvantages of the most common running surfaces and covers how to run safely on all of them.

Safety First

No matter where you run, you're going to run into trouble if you don't follow a few basic safety rules. Mind you, running isn't like rock climbing, where one false step can put an end to your career. As a runner, most of your safety concerns have to do with watching out for others. Unfortunately, daydreaming drivers and preying pouncers are part of our world.

Try to follow these basic personal safety guidelines for runners at all times:

➤ Always run facing traffic. When you're on roads, run defensively; assume that no driver sees you.

➤ Try to run with others. If you run alone, try to run where others are, such as parks, neighborhoods, or tracks.

➤ When you leave to run, tell someone where you'll be running and how long you plan to be out.

➤ Don't run the same route at the same time every day. Doing so makes it easier for someone to plan an attack.

➤ Know where phones, friendly homes, and open businesses are along your routes in case of an emergency.

➤ If you're verbally harassed, ignore it. Responding usually just spurs the sickos on.

Rules of the Road
You'll see a lot of runners wearing portable headphones. Don't be one of them. When you run wearing headphones, you're surrendering one of your main ways of staying alert. You won't be able to hear cars and potential bad guys. Save the music for getting psyched to run beforehand or for relaxing afterward.

➤ Be extra alert near thick bushes and other places where attackers can hide.

➤ If you're set upon by a dog, stop. If it persists, yell at it firmly. It will usually run away. Don't count on being able to outrun it.

➤ If you're set upon by an unarmed human, create as much of a commotion as possible, and try to escape. If the assailant is armed, don't resist, but try to get a good description to give to the police.

I know this sounds like a lot to keep in mind. And it sure seems as though always being concerned about safety will take a lot of the fun out of running. But there are some strange people out there. Being on guard for them is better than letting them really ruin your running by having their way.

Road Warriors

Now that that unpleasantness is out of the way, let's look at where you should run. The most common place to run, and usually the most convenient, is the road. Most people can just step outside of their homes, hit the road, and be off on an infinite number of routes.

The three main types of routes that runners use are *loops, out-and-backs,* and *point-to-points. Loops* involve running a big circuit around your starting and finishing point. *Out-and-backs* are where you head out for a set time or distance, usually with just a few turns, turn around at halfway, and then retrace your steps home. With a *point-to-point* route, you start at one place and end at another. This type of route usually requires someone to drop you off or meet you at one end.

Roads are good places to run because you're usually familiar with the ones in your neighborhood. A lot of times, running in known territory makes a run go by more quickly mentally. The firm footing of most asphalt road surfaces means that you don't have to worry about turning an ankle, as you might if you're running on grass or rugged trails. Races are almost always going to be held on roads, so by training on them, you'll be used to that surface if you decide that you want to race. Roads are also a good choice because you can drive courses in your car before running on them so that you know what the footing, terrain, and distance will be like.

Of course, that firm footing comes with a price. Humans didn't evolve to run for hours at a time on asphalt. If you're new to running, you're probably going to be sore enough for the first couple of months. Pounding away on a hard surface will probably only make that soreness worse. That's why it's so important to have a good pair of running shoes if you're going to be taking it to the streets. (For more on running shoes, see Chapter 7, "Sole Mates: Finding the Right Running Shoe.")

Another thing to be mindful of on the roads is the slant. Most roads tilt slightly from the center. If you're running against traffic, your left leg will be operating as if it's a bit longer than your right one. Also, your right foot will turn in a bit more when you land because you're on an uneven surface. Both of these stresses to your legs can lead to injury, so try to avoid roads that have a really obvious slant to them. Run toward the middle of the road if you can safely do so.

And let's not forget our good friend, the automobile. Regardless of what traffic laws say about sharing the roads, cars rule. Thanks to the millions of runners out there, things are definitely better than they were 25 years ago, when runners on the roads were looked upon as freaks. Today, at least, most drivers are used to seeing runners on a regular basis, but that doesn't mean that they're going to cut you much slack. The solution?

> **Training Tip**
> Devise your running loops with smaller loops in mind. That way, if you run into trouble or just don't feel up to your original plans for the day, you can cut your run short.

Training Tip
Most runners have a few standard routes they do on a regular basis. Being on a course you're used to can make the miles go by faster because you'll have a better idea of how far you have to go and can dole out your effort accordingly. On days when you need variety, feel free to explore.

Do your best to stay off of heavily traveled roads. Even in the busiest cities, you can usually find a mile or two of relatively open road. In addition to being safer, less-traveled roads are just a lot more fun to run on because you can relax a bit more and feel a bit more like you're getting away from it all.

Although they're not really roads, I'll include bike paths in this section also because they're usually made of asphalt. Don't let the name fool you. Runners know that "bike path" is usually code for "nice place to run where you don't have to worry about cars." In Boston, for example, there's an asphalt path along both sides of the Charles River for about nine miles in each direction. It's where most of Boston's runners congregate to get in some hassle-free miles away from busy streets. Most metropolitan areas have at least a few miles of bike paths. Seek them out.

Run Away from Sidewalks

There's not much to say about running on sidewalks other than that you should avoid it whenever possible. Sure, sidewalks are safer than roads with respect to cars, and maybe they don't feel all that much different from asphalt. But they're made from concrete and cement, which are some of the hardest surfaces around. When you figure that with every running step, you subject your body to a force equal to at least three times your body weight, it should be obvious that you want to do whatever you can to lower that impact shock.

Rules of the Road
When you're overtaking walkers or other runners, especially on a narrow path, alert them by saying, "On your left" when you're a few steps away from passing them. Otherwise, they might be startled if you suddenly breeze by them.

Another good reason to avoid running on sidewalks is that they seldom provide an uninterrupted surface for long. You're continually going up and down, up and down for driveways and curbs. This unevenness only adds to the pounding on your legs and is a good way to twist an ankle, too.

The only time it's worth clinging to sidewalks is when you're running in a busy section of a city. Even then, though, you'll probably be making your way to a park, bike path, or other better option for the bulk of your run. Otherwise, try to spend as little time running on sidewalks as possible.

Lap It Up: Tracks

Another of the most popular and obvious places to run is on a track. Its plusses are many:

➤ You can easily track (so to speak) your distance and/or pace, giving you a quantifiable means of monitoring your progress.

➤ You can stop immediately if something goes wrong.

➤ You're usually in a safe, secure area. Many tracks are lit for an hour or two in the evening in the winter.

➤ There are no cars to deal with.

➤ There are no hills to deal with.

➤ You often have easy access to water fountains and bathrooms.

➤ You don't have to worry about potholes, hidden roots, and other things that can trip you on roads or trails.

Add to these advantages the fact that synthetic and rubberized tracks transmit about 20 percent less shock to your legs than asphalt does, and you can see why so many runners, especially beginners, find the track to be a safe haven. Another nice thing about outdoor tracks is that they're standardized. Almost all tracks at high schools in the United States are 400 meters around. If you didn't pay attention in school when the metric system was discussed, don't worry. One mile equals 1,609 meters. So four laps of a 400-meter track is 1,600 meters, just nine meters (roughly 30 feet) short of a mile. It takes you only a few seconds to run nine meters, so do what most runners do: ignore the difference, and count four laps of an outdoor track as a mile.

Rules of the Road

When you're running on the track, it's common runner's etiquette to cede the inside lanes to faster runners. If you hear someone from behind you yell, "Track!" that means to move to the outside to let them through.

Footnotes

Today, near the beginning of the 21st century, most outdoor tracks are 400 meters long because of what happened in the 19th century. Back then, the tracks in England, which is considered the pacesetter for modern track and field, were a quarter-mile around, which is 440 yards. But when Frenchman Pierre du Corbertin began to push for the Olympics to be revived in the late 1890s, England wanted to be in sync with the rest of Europe, and the yard tracks were converted to metric distances to standardize measurement.

The biggest problem with running on a track is the tedium. I know I start feeling like a caged rat sometimes if I'm just running around and around on a track at an easy pace. Most runners find that running for more than half an hour on a track starts to get on their nerves. One way around this problem is to run with a friend in the outside lanes. The time will pass a lot more quickly if you're talking away with a buddy by your side.

Track Talk
If you see someone running hard on the track for a lap at a time, he or she is doing *quarters*. They're called this because even though most tracks are measured metrically, runners usually ignore the small difference in distance and figure that four laps equals one mile. One lap, then, is a quarter of a mile.

Training Tip
If you're doing a distance run on the track, switch directions every mile. This switching will help you to keep track of your distance and will evenly distribute the stress of leaning into the curves to both of your hips. To further reduce that stress, run in the outside lanes, where the turns aren't as tight.

Another way to beat boredom on the track is to try to lose track of the number of laps you've run. Just like when you're running a new route on the roads, run for your usual amount of time, and figure that you'll cover roughly your usual distance.

Most long-time runners go to a track only when they want to do their one or two hard workouts of the week. During these workouts, they want to be on the track because they can precisely gauge their effort. They'll go to the track with a set workout in mind (such as doing *quarters*) and watch every second to make sure they're sticking to their plan as closely as possible. (For more on these types of workouts, see Chapter 19.) Why don't they run on the track most days? Because one of the greatest pleasures of running is exploring nature and enjoying a variety of scenery and terrain. Despite all of its other benefits, the track doesn't offer that variety.

Lack of variety is part of the reason that most long-time runners avoid indoor tracks. It can be pretty tough to get in runs of any real length on the indoor tracks that you'll find in the United States. Most of them require at least 10 laps just to cover one mile. I know this feeling all too well. When I started running again in the early '70s, I ran mostly at an indoor track at the YMCA. Around and around and around I ran. Next thing I knew, I had covered half a mile. So once I felt a bit more confident about my running, I moved outside and rediscovered how much more fun it is to run in the great outdoors. (I'll cover the other indoor running option, treadmills, in Chapter 9.)

The other good reason to use indoor tracks only when you have to is that they're so small that the turns are very tight. Even more than standard outdoor tracks do, these indoor tracks place undue strain on the hip facing the inside of the track.

The Off-Road Option

Run on soft surfaces such as dirt, grass, or trails made of crushed stone, cinders, or wood chips as much as possible. These are the types of forgiving ground that, as a species, humans grew up running over. Think about how much more pleasant it feels on your feet to walk across your yard than it does to walk down the street. Multiply that difference not only by the much greater pounding of running, but also by the thousands of steps that you take in a run, and you reach the unavoidable conclusion that running on natural surfaces is one of the best ways to avoid injury.

When I was in college, I did a lot of my running on trails, and I loved it. There's something psychologically soothing about cruising through the woods. You're likely to feel more relaxed during and after your run than if you're always having to worry about whether a car is going to come tearing around the next bend. A lot of trails are shaded, too, so you stay cooler and aren't subject to the sun's rays.

Footnotes

The Rails to Trails Conservancy converts old railroad lines into multiuse recreational paths. These are great places to run—they're free of auto traffic, they're usually scenic and have a soft surface, and they're always flat. The Conservancy currently administers more than 900 trails throughout the country, for more than 9,000 miles of running room. To find one near you, visit the organization's World Wide Web site (www.railtrails.org) or call it at (202) 331-9696.

Finding convenient trails to run on can be tricky. Check with local hiking clubs and horse stables for sites in your area. And don't feel guilty about driving to a trail for a run. People drive to parks to sit around and eat hot dogs, so what's the harm in taking a short trip for a satisfying run in the woods?

Even if you can't run on trails on a regular basis, you can still reduce the pounding on your legs by seeking out soft surfaces wherever you are. I usually try to run on the small strip of dirt or grass by the side of a road rather than on the asphalt. Soon after I turned 40, I stopped doing this, figuring that with my ever-advancing age, I needed as sure a footing as I could get. Well, guess what happened? Soon after switching from the dirt and grass to the roads, I had my first real injury in years. Now, I'm back to the side of the road whenever possible.

Rules of the Road

If you drive to a trail or park to run, bring dry clothes and fluids for after the run. That way, you can drive home comfortably and therefore more safely.

I originally made that switch away from dirt and grass because the footing on softer surfaces can be a bit tricky. Holes, roots, and uneven patches are a lot harder to see than on a hard road or track. In my high school days, I once cut the bottom of my feet by running across broken glass that I couldn't see on the ground. And some trails, no matter how mentally soothing, are just too rugged for most runners to be able to maintain their normal stride.

Nonetheless, I remain convinced that all runners benefit from running on smooth natural surfaces. Most of the best runners in the world, such as the Kenyans and Ethiopians, do the bulk of their mileage on dirt roads and trails. This training strengthens their leg muscles and tendons, and when they get on the roads, they can fly. The same will be true for you. Beginning runners, who might be heavier than veteran runners, will really benefit from the reduced pounding they get when running on soft surfaces.

Reach the Beach

I used to run a 10K (6.2 miles) race on the beach in Duxbury, Massachusetts every year. This beach was a firm, flat surface on which I could pretty much run with my normal stride. In other words, it was unlike most beaches. Despite what you might see on *Baywatch* or *Chariots of Fire*, there's just not that much good running to be had on the sand. Most beaches are either too soft, so that your feet sink too far into the sand with every step to run normally, or, by the time you get to firm footing near the water, they're too slanted. In the latter case, you're asking for the same type of trouble as when you run on a slanted road.

There are exceptions, and some runners find a certain mystical element in running by the ocean when the footing is good. On the central California coast, there's a place called Pismo Beach. (If it sounds familiar, that might be because that's one of the places that Bugs Bunny was always claiming that he had taken a wrong turn at.) The sand at Pismo Beach is ideal for running. It's flat and firm for about 50 yards from the water's edge. I know a runner who has done two-hour runs there, finding great joy in watching and listening to the crashing of the surf just feet away. If you can find one of these rare runable beaches, they're a nice treat, although even the most Zen-like runner would find them boring on a daily basis.

Outer Destinations

Now that we've looked at where to run when you're in familiar surroundings, let's look at what happens when you're a stranger in a strange land. A lot of beginning runners, no matter how committed they are when at home, blow off their running when they're traveling for business or pleasure. That's a shame. You know how running is such a stress reliever in your day-to-day life. It's that much more of one when you're away from your usual routine. Plus, running in a new town or city allows you to experience it in a way that you can't if you confine yourself to meeting rooms, tour buses, and restaurants.

Finding good places to run when you're traveling can be difficult. Most inactive people don't have a good sense of distance. If you ask them where to run, they might mention a local park and not realize that it's not quite going to fit your running needs because it's only 100 yards across. Or they might know of a large enough place to run, but because it's a mile or two away, they'll think that it might as well be on Mars as far as being accessible.

As with other aspects of travel, a good solution is to do some investigation before you leave home. Contact the local running clubs or running stores. If you can, do this before you make lodging reservations. When I'm in New York City, I always make sure that my hotel is no more than half a mile from Central Park, which is really the only place in Manhattan to get in some unimpeded miles.

These days, most cities have set aside some land for recreational purposes. It might not be great running, it might not be more than a mile or so of ground, and it probably won't be as beautiful as Central Park, but it can be the difference between being able to run and not. Besides parks, one common place to run is along waterfronts, such as along Lake Michigan in Chicago.

Training Tip

When you arrive in an unfamiliar locale, always look for uncomplicated places to run. Keep an eye out for bike paths, parks, and other places that will have at least a mile or two of open space so that you won't have to risk getting lost or remembering routes that involve tons of turns.

Footnotes

The American Running and Fitness Association maintains running maps for more than 200 U.S. cities. You can call them at (800) 776-ARFA. The e-mail address is listed in Appendix B, but for running map service, they prefer phone calls.

Don't forget that one of the keys to successful traveling is adaptability. This is as true with regard to running as it is to plane departures. If no good running options present themselves, make the most out of the hand you're dealt. When I was in postwar Vietnam a few years ago, the only place I could find to run without being overrun by traffic was a 600-yard loop through a zoo. This was hardly ideal, but circling that loop seemingly endlessly was a lot better than not running at all. In this country, if nothing else, you can usually find an outdoor track by looking for the nearest high school or college.

The Least You Need to Know

➤ No matter where you're running, the key to running safely is to be on constant guard for threats from cars, dogs, and suspicious humans.

➤ Streets and tracks are the most common and convenient places to run, but they have their drawbacks: streets are hard and can be dangerous, and tracks can be boring.

➤ The best place to run to avoid injury is on soft natural surfaces, especially dirt trails.

➤ Sidewalks and beaches are rarely good places to run.

➤ When you're traveling, you can find good places to run by calling local running clubs or running stores.

Morning, Noon, or Night: When to Run

There's a guy in the Washington, DC area who is known to some as Busy Running Man. That's because when he's spotted on the roads, he's running while wearing headphones and, incredibly, reading the morning newspaper. Is he an expert at maximizing the effectiveness of his time, having figured out how to do three things at once? Or is he among the world's worst at managing his time, always having to cram too many activities into too small an amount of time?

I tend toward the latter view. I say that because Busy Running Man seems to exemplify (admittedly in exaggerated form) what so many people think about running: so much is going on in their lives that it's a constant struggle to find the time for it. "I don't have the time" is the most frequent excuse that people give for not exercising regularly. That's almost never true. In this chapter, I'll show you how to find the time to fit running into your schedule, as well as detail the benefits of working out at various times of the day.

Fitting It in Your Schedule

Training Tip
People who think they don't have time to run because their day consists of running from one responsibility to another should consider this: In the average American home, the television is on for seven hours a day. Bypass one roundup of the latest local mayhem and one repeat of *Seinfeld*, and you've got more than enough time to get in a good workout.

As I said, a lack of time is the reason most often cited when people are asked why they don't exercise regularly. You're reading this book, so I'm not going to lump you into the always-looking-for-an-excuse category. What you want to know is where to find the time. But let's look at these people's claim nonetheless, if for no other reason than to keep you motivated if you hit a snag in your running program and start to think that your busy life means that your fitness must be sacrificed.

Running Out of Time?

Usually, people who say that they don't have time for exercise have never made it a part of their life. They don't understand what it means to feel fit, so they don't place any importance on it. They've been taught that exercise is always drudgery, and they think that their life is hard enough as it is. Why would they take precious time to make it more so? Also, they think that they're already so tired all the time. Why run, and get more tired?

What U.S. Presidents Know That You Don't

Almost all of the 8 million regular runners in the United States are very busy. They hold demanding jobs; they're parents; they volunteer in their communities. But they know that the tiny amount of time that it takes each week to stick with a running program gives them a return that is monumental. The physical and psychological strength that they get from running increases the amount of "time" in their lives, if you take "time" to mean hours in which they feel vibrant, productive, and at ease with themselves.

Let's look at it another way and break things down mathematically: There are 168 hours in a week. You can maintain a good level of fitness by running for half an hour, four times a week. So there's two hours. Throw in another 15 minutes each workout for stretching, cooling down, and so on, and you're up to a grand total of three hours out of every week's 168.

Can't find three hours? Life too busy? Consider the U.S. President, who, it's generally agreed, has the busiest, most difficult job in the world. Of our last four presidents, three—Bill Clinton, George Bush, and Jimmy Carter—have been regular runners. They all know how running centers their day and increases the quality of the rest of their time.

Footnotes

Jimmy Carter knew the value of setting aside time for running long before he became president. He was a member of the cross-country team while a student at the Naval Academy. Michael Dukakis, who unsuccessfully ran for Carter's former job in 1988, also came to politics with a running history. In 1951, he finished 57th at the Boston Marathon in 3 hours, 31 minutes.

None of this information is meant to belittle your busy life. It *is* a struggle to find the time to run regularly. I just wanted to make sure that you're convinced that it's a worthwhile struggle, and one that can almost always be won. Here are some ways to manage your running time so that it easily becomes a regular part of your day:

➤ Consider your run an integral part of your day, as you do going to work and spending time with your family.

➤ When planning your day, plan when you're going to run. Don't expect the time to magically present itself.

➤ Treat running as an extension of your work day. Don't consider yourself "done for the day" until you've gotten your run in.

➤ Instead of viewing running as another responsibility, look upon your running time as a gift to yourself each day, when you get to spend quiet, quality time by yourself or with a close friend or two.

➤ Plan runs with friends one or two days a week. Give these meetings the same degree of commitment as you do other meetings during the week.

➤ Explain to your family and friends the specialness of this time to you. They'll be more likely to respect and support your running if you share with them why it's so important.

➤ If necessary, schedule your runs the same way that you do other parts of your life. Write them on a calendar or leave yourself a note.

Training Tip

It takes a lot less work to maintain fitness than to acquire it. You can cut your training to just one-third its usual level for a few weeks and not really lose any aerobic capacity. So if your schedule gets uncharacteristically hectic for brief periods, schedule just a few short runs a week, and you won't have to worry about starting from scratch when things return to normal.

Above all, keep a flexible approach rather than an all-or-nothing attitude. When things seem out of control at work, you don't just blow it off and head home for the day. You adapt to the situation and do the best you can. If work or other responsibilities has cut into the start of your usual running time, don't consider the day lost, and not run at all. If anything, you'll need running's stress relief more than usual. So get out the door for whatever amount of time is left to you. Then look at the time-consuming situation and see whether it's avoidable next time.

Morning Glory

The best time to run is the time of day when your normal schedule will most regularly allow you to run. For many busy people, that time is the morning. Studies of adult exercisers have shown the highest rate of regular compliance among those who work out is in the morning. It's no surprise why—other than the sandman, there usually aren't a whole lot of people placing demands on you at 6 a.m. But come the end of the work day, you might be pulled a million different ways, and it might be a lot easier to justify missing a run than to have to say "no" to people.

Rules of the Road
Air pollution levels are lowest in the morning. When there's serious smog going on, all runners should consider switching to morning runs. Even in less severe conditions, asthmatics and others with respiratory problems will breathe easier if they do at least their summer running early in the day. (They'll also stay cooler.)

Most regular morning runners find that hitting the roads before work or school gives them energy for the whole day. It sure beats staggering out of bed at the last minute and starting your day in a stupor behind the wheel. Mentally, there are few greater feelings than starting your work day knowing that you've already achieved something personally significant.

Morning runners should take some extra precautions, however. Some studies have shown that regular morning runners get injured more often than evening runners. Your muscles are stiffer in the morning, and it's harder to feel as though you're making a smooth transition from rest to activity in the morning, especially when going right into a *wake-up run*. Additionally, most of the physiological attributes that contribute to good distance running, such as aerobic capacity, peak in the late afternoon and early evening, so you have to work a little harder in the morning to maintain a given pace. Also, most morning runners are trying to squeeze in a run without being late for work, so they might tend to skimp on a proper warm-up. You can see why morning runners might get injured more easily.

Track Talk
Some runners stumble out of bed and almost right into a *wake-up run*. This type of run just covers a few miles at an easy pace to get your body revved up for the rest of the day. Usually, wake-up runs aren't a runner's main workout of the day.

But that doesn't mean you have to get injured. The solution is to include time for some gentle stretching, and just some overall waking up, when you're setting your alarm clock for the next morning's run. Give yourself at least 20 minutes from when you get out of bed to when you get out the door. Thirty minutes would be even better.

I know that this is precious time seemingly taken away from sleep. There are two things you can do to counter that feeling. First, if your entire wake-up/warm-up/run/cool-down routine is going to take an hour, then go to bed an hour earlier the night before. (Try not to do it the other way and get up an hour earlier than usual after going to bed at your normal time.) But what about all that stuff you need to do in the evening before you go to bed? My second bit of time-management advice is to save some of the little chores, such as paying a couple of bills or packing lunches, for that wake-up time I advise between getting out of bed and starting your run. If you've ever started the day by running as a beautiful sunrise unfolds, you know that the effort of getting out of bed is usually worth it.

The Lunch Bunch

Another of the main when-to-run options is the middle of the day. When I was training for the 1976 Olympics, I was employed as a teacher. Running before and after school every day was starting to get to me, so I asked for and received permission to run during my lunch hour. This was a huge help. It broke up my work day, gave me a boost for the afternoon, and allowed me to get in a better quality workout than when I was continually dragging myself out of bed to run. (I'm not much of a morning person.)

Running at lunchtime is also nice because, as with morning running, you have the post-work hours free to spend with family and friends. During the winter, running in the middle of the day often can be your only chance for any real sunlight until the weekends. This is also usually the warmest time of day in the winter. (It is in the summer, too, when it can be a good idea to look for a different time of day to run.)

The biggest problem you're going to face as a noon-time runner is logistics. Your employers might not see the value in you dashing out the door every day for a vigorous run, especially if they're not exercisers and think that you're going to spend the afternoon asleep at your desk. That's why it's a good idea to do what I did and discuss your desire to run at lunch with your boss. As you should with your family, explain why this time is important to you. (You could also hit them with the statistics that show that the fittest employees take the fewest number of sick days.)

Training Tip
Carbohydrates ingested within 30 minutes of finishing a run are absorbed three times quicker than otherwise. This fuel replenishes your muscles and speeds your recovery from run to run, so don't let a tight pre-work schedule prevent you from getting something in your system between finishing a morning run and going to the office.

Training Tip
If you're going to run in the middle of a work day, start preparing for it about 15 minutes before your lunch hour. Stand up at your desk and do some gentle stretching of your back, neck, shoulders, and legs. This stretching will ease the transition from being an office stiff to a flowing runner.

You might need more than the standard time allotted for lunch in your company to get in your run. It's not in your long-term best interest to sprint out the door at 12:01, return at 12:56 and be back, dressed, at your desk at 1:01. Account for the necessary pre- and post-run activities as you should when planning a run in the morning. Present your boss with a good plan, such as taking an extra 30 minutes in the middle of the day in exchange for arriving earlier or staying later.

After getting the thumbs up from your boss, you're going to have to assess the surroundings. The number of businesses that have showers on site is growing, but they're still rare. Check for health clubs near your office at which you can stretch and shower afterward. If reasonable, this option is often a good one for helping to maintain your professional identity—you'll leave and return to work in your office attire, rather than your coworkers seeing you in shorts and a T-shirt.

When there's not an accessible shower, some runners towel off in the bathroom. This is a judgment call, based on your preferences, as well as the degree of formality of your office and the closeness of contact with your coworkers. Let's just say I wouldn't want to be around some runners a couple of hours after they've run if they had yet to shower.

Track Talk
Doubling is running twice during a day. Ambitious recreational runners, as well as most professional runners, do a run in the morning, and then run again in the afternoon or evening. Usually, one run is about twice as long as the other.

Training Tip
One way to combine your running with your home responsibilities is to run with your dog. It can get its needed exercise and bathroom trips, and you can cross two things off your daily to-do list at once.

Night Training

Hit the roads after a stressful day, and by the end of the run, you start to entertain the possibility that perhaps your boss only *seems* to be the devil incarnate. Even if you feel tired from a long work day, you usually feel better after you've warmed up when you run in the evening than at any other time of the day. Getting out for some miles after work is also a wonderful way to separate your professional life from your personal life. Some runners swear by their late afternoon/early evening runs even if they have already had a morning or noontime run. They get tremendous energy from this *doubling*.

But consistently getting in your runs after work can be tough if you're not dedicated. You're seldom going to get a call early in the morning from your boss asking you to come in two hours early, but the same isn't true when it comes to staying late at the office. If you have a family, they might be in the reasonable, even endearing habit of wanting to spend time with you when you get home from work, rather than watch you dart out the door in your running shoes. There's also the matter of holding up others' mealtimes to consider.

Having someone to run with right after work can help mightily in sticking with it. It's often easier to find running partners for the afternoon, when people tend to be congregated in fewer areas, than in the morning, when you're scattered all over the place. Another solution is to start your run from your office. By the time you've finished your run, the traffic will be lighter, and you can go home and devote your entire attention to what's waiting for you there.

Weekend Warriors

As I said in Chapter 3, "Taking Your First Steps," you want to progress intelligently with your running. That usually doesn't mean doing most of your running for the week on the consecutive days of the weekend. But that's what you'll see a lot of time-pressed runners do, figuring that they'll trash themselves on Saturday and Sunday and then have the work week to recoup and do it all again the next weekend. That's not a good approach unless one of your main goals as a runner is to get injured.

Still, if it's always a major effort to find the time to run during the work week, you can use the weekends to your advantage. Say you're running four days a week. Have Saturday and Sunday be two of those days. That means you only have to squeeze in two runs between Monday and Friday. Just be sure to plan intelligently. It's usually best to do your weekend running in the mornings. You can still sleep in some, go for a nice run, enjoy breakfast with your family, and then have hours free for whatever else you want to do.

One time-honored running tradition is to do the longest run of the week on the weekend. The runs before and after that longest run should be relatively short, easy runs. So you could go for a short run Saturday morning, still have almost the entire day for other activities, and then do your longest run for the week on Sunday morning. The short run on Saturday is just a warm-up to loosen you up for Sunday's run. Or you could do your long run on Saturday and find a little time on Sunday for a short run that will help to work out the kinks from the previous day's effort.

Running Here and There

The more convenient that you can make your running, the better. That's why some busy runners try to combine it with other parts of their lives when possible. For example, you leave your car with the mechanic for repairs, and rather than bother a friend to follow you there, you run home. Or you spend a full day with the family at a mall or at a park and have your spouse drop you off a few miles from home on the return trip. Obviously, these aren't everyday solutions, but if your life is as busy as most people's, it can help to always be thinking of ingenious ways to squeeze in runs or catch a *quick-few*. These out-of-the-ordinary jaunts are sometimes among the most fun.

> **Track Talk**
> If there are a lot of demands on your time on a given day, but you want to sneak out of the house for a run, tell others that you're just doing a *quick-few*. This is what you say to family and friends to try to fool them that you're going to be gone for so little time that they'll hardly notice that you're gone.

A more routine example of this kind of thinking is running to and from work. My co-author, Scott Douglas, used to do this when he lived a few miles from his office and really came to look forward to it. Scott would run home from work on, say, Monday night, lengthening the basic route by however much he wanted. When he got home, he enjoyed the feeling of being done with both work and running for the day. It didn't hurt that his commute via foot didn't take all that much more time than by car. The next morning, Scott would run to work. Knowing that your car is at the office is a pretty good incentive to get in a morning run! There, Scott would shower and change into the work clothes that he had brought in on the previous day. Sure sounds better than sitting in a traffic jam.

The Least You Need to Know

➤ Almost everyone has enough time in their schedules for a regular running program.

➤ A good running program need only take 3 hours out of the 168 hours in a week.

➤ The best time to run is whatever time of day you'll consistently have the fewest demands on your time.

➤ Plan for and set aside your running time the same way that you plan other important parts of your life.

➤ Busy adults tend to have the highest compliance rates when they run in the morning.

Chapter 6

Mo' Better Motivation

In This Chapter

➤ Developing good goals to stay motivated

➤ Setting the right types of goals

➤ Keeping written records of your running

➤ Running with others to stay motivated

Ask runners who have been running for six months or more if they hope to run for the rest of their lives, and almost all of them are going to say yes. That's the easy part—recognizing that your life is better because you run. What's not so easy is knowing how to stay motivated enough along the way to keep running.

Inertia is a mighty powerful force, and it can be tough to keep in mind how much better running makes you feel. So it can be difficult to resist that little voice that tells you that your life is hard enough as it is, so you just can't deal with running this week. Then one week becomes two, then three, and then you're way off track.

In this chapter, I'll show you some basic motivational strategies that I and other long-time runners use to keep ourselves on the road. If you get in the habit of using a few of the methods I tell you about here, not only will you want to run for the rest of your life, but you'll be psychologically able to.

Beyond the Basics

What I have to say in this chapter applies to all runners, whether you've made one trip around the block or have run so many miles that you could circle the globe. That said, I'm going to focus in this chapter on what I call "Phase Two" runners. By that I mean runners who have already successfully taken that hardest initial step, from inactivity to regular running. These runners have achieved that basic level of fitness that I showed you how to reach in Chapter 3. But having reached that, they might very well think, "What now?"

After all, when you're new to running, you probably don't always find the running itself easy, but keeping at it is in some ways easier because it's so foreign to you. When you follow a moderate progression like the one I outlined in Chapter 3, you can see gains almost from run to run. It's hard not to be motivated when from week to week you see that you can run farther, that running is becoming easier, that you're losing weight, feeling better, and so on. This period can be one of the most exciting times in your running life.

You know that you feel better than when you started running. But how do you keep at it? How do you make the leap to where you look at running as something that grounds, not interrupts, your day? How do you stay motivated?

Goal for It!

This book contains more than 100,000 words. That's a lot of writing! How do you go about tackling such a big project? You set intermediate goals and then set short-term goals to get you to those intermediate goals. You track your progress toward these short-term goals, all the while reminding yourself of the long-term goal, and when necessary and appropriate, you review what you've done to remind yourself how far you've come. That's the approach that I recommend for running as well. You need to set both short-term and long-term goals, you need a way to track those goals, and you need to monitor how you're progressing toward your goals, both to see whether they need to be revised and to remind yourself how far you've come.

For most runners, the ultimate long-term goal is to keep running for the rest of their lives. That's a pretty heady goal, and one that's hard to pin down. It's certainly my ultimate goal, but it's so vague that I can't use it as my main source of motivation. I set goals for a given year, and then within that year I set intermediate goals of what to focus on for a few months at a time. Within those few months, I set even shorter-term goals to guide me through a week or so of running at a time. Along the way, I'm constantly assessing things to determine what adjustments I need to make.

Again, consider this book. When I started to write it, I would have been lost if I would have said, "OK, I'm going to write more than 100,000 words about running. Let's get going!" Instead, I looked at finishing each chapter as a goal unto itself and finishing each section of each chapter as an even more immediate goal. Along the way, I'd monitor how

I was progressing. (Usually not as much as I'd like!) By plugging away like that, I was able to produce what you're reading now. You probably take this approach with your work as well without even thinking about it.

Keep It Real

To use goals to motivate you to run, start by setting short-term goals that you can achieve within three months. These goals should be specific and challenging, yet within your grasp. For example, your goal might be to be able to run three miles in less than 30 minutes at the end of three months. This goal is analogous to writing a chapter for this book.

Footnotes

Goals can take many forms. One of my first goals when I started running again in the '70s was to quit smoking. I set daily goals, such as smoking no more than five cigarettes in a day. The more I ran, the less I wanted to smoke, and the easier these goals became to reach.

To get to your short-term goal, you need to set shorter-term goals that follow a logical progression. After all, if you can now run two miles at a pace of 12 minutes per mile, and you keep doing that for the next 12 weeks, then you probably won't achieve your goal of three miles in 30 minutes. You need to map out intermediate steps along the way to get you from your starting point to your goal. To continue my writing analogy, those short-term steps are the sections within a chapter. The first section leads to the second section, which builds to the third section, and so on until a chapter is complete.

Your intermediate goals should be two to three months away so that you can achieve several shorter-term goals. Two to three months is long enough for you to make some progress in your running and long enough to allow for the setbacks that all runners encounter occasionally. But it's also a short enough period of time that you can stay focused on the goal.

Being specific with your goals is the best way to make sure that you can track your progress. "I'd like to run faster" or "I'd like to lose weight" are amorphous goals. Three weeks into your running program, you're probably running faster, and if you've lost a pound, then you've lost weight. So why continue? But if you

Training Tip

Your goals should be attainable with a reasonable amount of work, but they should be challenging. If your goals are too easy to reach, you're more likely to get bored with your running.

say, "I want to run three miles in less than 30 minutes by the end of June," or "I want to lose 10 pounds by the beginning of November," then you have something quantifiable to go after. You can chart a course toward meeting that goal, you can monitor your progress as you near it, and you can definitively say whether you achieved it.

Footnotes

In 1964, American Billy Mills wrote "Olympic gold; 28:24" on a piece of paper that he tacked to a wall. He looked at this paper every day while preparing for the Olympic 10K. Despite having a best time of only 29:10 before the Games, Mills ran with the best runners in the world in the Olympic final and won the gold medal in the last 100 yards. His time? 28:24.

The Means to Get to the Ends

The other big reason to be specific with your goals is because doing so will help you to know what to do to meet your goals. I turned 50 while writing this book. One of my big goals for my first year as a 50-year-old is to break the American record for 10 miles for a man of my age. That time is 52:24, which is just a bit faster than 5:15 per mile. So I know that I need to do some training at or faster than that pace to reach that goal. Contrast that goal with if I just said that I wanted to run a fast time for 10 miles. What does that mean? How fast? How would I know what to shoot for in my training?

Rules of the Road
You should write down your goals, but you shouldn't view them as being etched in stone. If you encounter an injury or other setback, but ignore it to keep working toward your goal, you'll only be setting yourself up for more setbacks. Only try to progress when you can do so healthfully; when you hit a physical setback, your goal should be to maintain, not improve, your fitness.

The same principles apply to your short-term goals. Do you want to be able to run five miles without stopping two months from now? OK, then you know that to get to that goal, you need to work up to three miles, then four miles, and so on at a pace that you can handle, rather than concentrating on how fast you're running.

When you meet that short-term, three-month goal, give yourself a break! Promise yourself a meaningful reward while you're working toward the goal, then give yourself that reward when you meet it. The reward could be a nice dinner at your spouse's expense, or a new piece of running apparel, or a book or CD that you've wanted for a long time.

Don't beat yourself up if you don't meet your goal. Instead, be honest about how much progress you made and evaluate why you didn't quite get to where you wanted. I might have a goal of running a certain time at an important race that's three months away. If I don't perform as well in the race as

I had wanted to, I pat myself on the back for what I did achieve in the race and then look at where and why I fell short. Did I set too tough of a goal? Was it unreasonable of me to expect to be at this point in three months based on my fitness when I started working toward the goal? Did I not work hard enough? Did I do the wrong types of things to get me to my goal?

Training Tip

Just as you shouldn't be intimidated by your goals, don't be limited by them either. If you reach a goal ahead of schedule, reward yourself, and then set a new, slightly tougher goal.

Ask these kinds of questions, and remember: You've almost undoubtedly made some progress. Say your goal was to be 15 pounds lighter at the end of three months, but you've lost 10 pounds. That's still a tremendous achievement! Focus on congratulating yourself for what you have done, not beating yourself up over where you might have fallen short. Then learn from your experience and move on toward your next goal.

Footnotes

If you need more help reaching your goals, check out *The Complete Idiot's Guide to Reaching Your Goals* by Jeff Davidson (Alpha Books, 1997). This book contains great tips and techniques for setting and achieving all of your goals.

Logging On

The best way to track your progress toward your goals is to keep a *training log*. This log is a notebook, journal, or even just random piles of paper in which you record key information about your running (see the following figure).

A training log gives you an objective record of your progress as a runner. A lot of runners, including me, regularly consult their training logs to look at the work they've done in the past to provide motivation for the future.

Track Talk

A *training log* is the place where you record important information about your running. You should keep some sort of training log because it allows you to monitor your progress and learn from your mistakes.

The changes that running causes are subtle on a day-to-day basis, and memories are notoriously selective. Taken together, those two things can make it hard to get a sense of how your running is going. But if you mark key information a few times a week in your log, you have an undeniable record.

When you're feeling down and thinking that you're not making any progress, you can look back and see that the run you just got back from that seemed to be a disaster would have been a major accomplishment just a few months ago. Many runners lack confidence in themselves and their abilities, and they downplay their accomplishments. By providing a visible manifestation of your running, training logs are great psychological comforters.

Keeping detailed records of your training allows you to better monitor your progress.

Your Very Own Guide Log

I like to use my training log to see how I'm chipping away at my goals. Say I'm aiming for that 10-mile race I talked about earlier. To get ready for that race, one of my key workouts is several repetitions of running hard for a mile, jogging very easily for a few minutes to recover, and then running hard again. As the race nears, I want to be sure that I'm doing the hard miles at least a few seconds a mile faster than the pace I hope to maintain in the race. After each workout, I write down my times for the hard miles. From week to week, I should be able to see that my times are improving. This record will motivate me to keep striving for my goal, or it can signal that I should revise my goal.

Use your log the same way. If your goal is to lose 20 pounds in the next four months, track your weight in your log. That's a goal that you can mark your progress to, just as focusing on a race and trying to reach a certain level of fitness for it is for me. The same principle applies if you've been running a few miles a day and want to try to run more. Write down with pride when you run farther than you have so you have a record of the great strides that you're making.

Training logs also help you to learn from your mistakes. Say that lately you've been dragging. Every run feels harder than it should, and you just don't seem to be as eager to run as usual. You look back in your log, and notice that a few weeks ago, you had the flu, but ran farther than usual anyway (runners are stubborn!). Training logs can help to remove some of the mystery from your running. Over time, you'll be able to see what does and doesn't work for you.

What to Write, When to Write

The more often you write in your training log, the more it can help you. Writing in your log within an hour of every run is ideal, because that's when the run is freshest in your mind. Another good time is soon before you go to bed, because you can put the run in perspective with the rest of the day. If you have a decent memory, it's OK not to write in your log after every run, but try to write in your log at least twice a week so that you don't forget to include relevant information.

What information should you include in your training log? It depends on what factors are significant to you in determining your progress. Here are just some of the things that runners record in their logs:

➤ Distance run

➤ How long the run took

➤ How the run felt subjectively

➤ What the course was like

➤ What the weather was like

➤ Any ache or pain during the run

➤ Whether the run was a solo effort or with others

➤ Weight

➤ Morning heart rate

➤ Number of hours slept

➤ Any other exercise for the day

➤ Significant nonrunning events that might make running harder or easier that day, such as a late night at work

➤ Mileage for the week and month

➤ Goal for the coming week and month

➤ Assessment of progress toward goals

Rules of the Road
Avoid the temptation to base your running around how impressive it will look in your log. If you're going to increase your mileage from week to week, do it because it will help you to meet a running goal, not just because it looks good in your log. Use your log as a tool to meet your goals rather than the source of your goals.

All of this information is more than most people want to write down a few times a week. At the minimum, I think you should include distance or time run, anything significant about the course or weather, anything significant about how you felt during the day or on the run, and, at least twice a month, how you're progressing toward your goals.

What you write in your training log might not seem important to anyone else in the world. No matter. One of the things I love most about running is that I do it solely for myself, and my success is determined solely by me. That kind of control is hard to achieve in most other areas of life. In running, there's no such thing as office politics, racial or gender discrimination, or other arbitrary things that can impede your progress. You can't schmooze your way into becoming a better runner. Your training log is a great place to turn to take refuge from these kinds of standards, because you can look in it and see the work you've done and the progress you've made. This clear reward for effort is hard to come by in most parts of our lives, even things that we're very passionate about, such as being a parent.

The Buddy System

The best way to stay motivated is to make your running interesting, easy, and enjoyable. The single best thing you can do to make your running easier and more enjoyable isn't getting the latest, greatest pair of shoes or eating just the right food, or putting on those cool running sunglasses. It's much simpler than that—run regularly with a friend. That person is your *training partner*.

Track Talk
A *training partner* is a runner of similar ability whom you run with on a regular basis.

We've all heard about the loneliness of the long-distance runner. Yes, running can be an intensely solitary experience, and that's one of the main things that many people love about it. I certainly enjoy the opportunity to get away from the usual distractions with only my thoughts to accompany me. But if that's how you always run, you're missing out on one of the greatest and generally unknown aspects of running—the social side. Most people find that the miles pass a lot quicker when they've got a friend by their side (see the following figure).

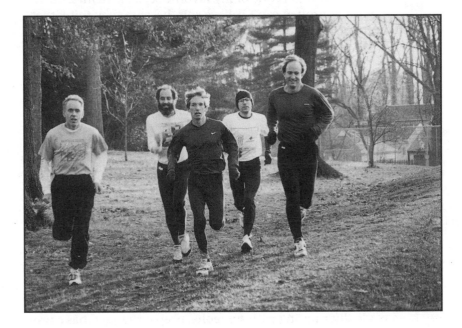

Running with friends of similar ability is the best way to make your running more enjoyable.

When I was training to be the best marathoner in the world in the '70s, I ran twice a day, pretty much every day of the year. That's a lot of runs! I had company on more than half of those runs. These days, I might run with someone else only once or twice a week. This makes the running tougher now, even though I only run about half the number of miles per year that I used to. That's because training partners are great motivators.

As I said in the introduction to this chapter, inertia can be one of your toughest foes as a runner. Once you get out the door and start running, you've won the battle for the day. The best way to do that is to plan to meet a friend to run. Knowing that your friend is depending on you to be at such and such place at such and such time makes it very unlikely that you won't show. Once you show up, you'll start your run, and the workout will take care of itself.

Training partners can also help to motivate you during your run. If the two of you have planned to run five miles together, but you're feeling a little apathetic that day, you're a lot more likely to stick with your original goal for the day when you're with someone than if you're running on your own. That's why even the most solitary runners often try to hook up with others for their longest run of the week.

In the same way, training partners can help you to get more out of yourself on days when you've planned to run faster than usual. You're just a lot less likely to give up and take it easy if you and a friend are out there sharing the effort, helping each other reach your potential.

Rules of the Road
It's OK to run occasionally with runners who are faster than you as a way to push yourself. But your regular training partners shouldn't be substantially faster than you, or you'll always be overdoing it. Conversely, if you regularly run with someone who is much slower than you, you'll be limiting your progress. A good rule of thumb is to try to find training partners who run within 30 seconds per mile of your normal pace.

Not that running with someone else is all about mutual teeth gritting and pain withstanding. Running at an easy pace with others is one of my favorite social activities. Nonrunners often can't believe this, because they think that running always hurts and always leaves you breathless. The opposite is usually true when you run with a friend—you can't get yourselves to shut up! For a lot of people, running seems to loosen their tongues like a few drinks do. (Note that when you run with someone else, you'll regularly be seeing whether you can pass the talk test and are running at the right level of effort.)

How do you find training partners? The easiest way is to have a friend or spouse who runs at about the same pace as you, but don't worry if you don't. Most local running clubs hold group runs a few times a week. There, runners of similar pace levels will hook up, even if they don't know each other. You can also meet potential training partners through the people who finish near you in a race.

I don't want to get too hokey here, but the whole idea of training partners is a big reason why I think runners lead more interesting lives than most people. Once you're an adult, it can be pretty tough to make new friends away from work. But running with someone, even a stranger, has a way of making bonds like few other things do. Running has created and strengthened innumerable friendships, because the training partners have been through so much together.

Avoid the Extremes

Consistency is the key to progressing as a runner. It's infinitely easier to stay motivated if you can see that you're able to steadily chip away at your goals. Try to avoid the extremes of overdoing it or not doing it.

Most of this chapter is about how to keep running. You want to know how to prevent those spells where you don't run for a week or two at a time and see your progress erode. Avoiding these spells is important because psychologically, periods of low motivation can feed on each other so that the less you run, the more frustrated you get, and the more you feel like giving up because your goals seem farther and farther away. Physically, it's important to keep at it because after as little as one week away from running, you start to lose the benefits. One study found that after only two to three weeks of inactivity, a group of runners lost almost half of their aerobic fitness. Talk about use it or lose it!

But consider the other extreme on the motivation scale. Runners are ambitious people; after all, no one is making you do this sometimes difficult thing. Just by starting a running program, you've shown that you are motivated. Problems can arise when that motivation runs amok. You can get so fired up that you start running more than you're ready for. In that case, you're *overtraining*. When that happens, you'll eventually either get injured or get so burned out that you won't want to run. In either case, you'll be as susceptible to seeing your fitness slip away as if you were undermotivated.

Overtraining is most common in highly ambitious runners who think that more miles are always better than fewer miles. They base their training more on reaching a certain number of miles per week than on structuring their training to best meet their goals. As a result, they wind up running a lot of *junk miles*. Also, they usually don't meet their goals, and they get injured and feel flat pretty easily.

Because the amount of running people can handle varies so much from individual to individual, overtraining can happen at what might seem like a low level of mileage. If you go from being sedentary to running 15 miles a week within a month, you're putting far more stress on your body than if you were a long-time runner who increased his or her mileage from 40 to 55 miles per week. Unfortunately, overtraining isn't like a broken leg, where you definitely know what's bothering you. Its symptoms are many, and they can be caused by a lot of things besides just running too much.

Still, there are some ways to determine whether you're overtrained or to prevent overtraining in the first place. One of the best ways is to regularly measure your *resting heart rate*, or pulse. Over the course of several mornings, see how many times your heart beats in one minute when you first wake. If possible, try to take your pulse on mornings when you don't wake to an alarm clock. Your resting heart rate is usually going to be within a few beats of the same measure from day to day.

Rules of the Road
Common runner's etiquette is to let the slowest member of a group set the pace, rather than everyone straining to keep up with the fastest member of the group.

Track Talk
Overtraining is running more than your body can handle for at least a few weeks. Overtraining can lead to injury and burnout. The amount of running that constitutes overtraining varies from runner to runner.

Track Talk
When you run more to get in a certain number of miles per week rather than to meet your goals, you're doing *junk miles*. This kind of running is just mindlessly accumulating miles, usually for the sake of having an impressive-looking training log.

Track Talk
The number of times that your heart beats in one minute when you're doing nothing is your *resting heart rate*. It's usually lowest in the morning when you're lying in bed, especially if you don't wake to an alarm clock.

If your resting heart rate is more than five beats per minute higher than usual, something's up. You might be on the verge of getting sick, or you might be dehydrated, or you might be under a lot of stress. For whatever reason, your heart has to work harder than usual just to maintain your body's systems at rest. If that's the case, then think how much harder than usual it's going to have to work when you run.

If your morning pulse remains elevated for a few consecutive days, you need to take it easy. If you're not sick, or can't otherwise explain why your pulse might be higher than usual, then you're on the verge of overtraining. If you keep running at your usual level, you are risking injury and staleness.

Other signs of overtraining are the following:

➤ No desire to run on most days

➤ Lower energy during the day and when you run

➤ "Heavy" legs that don't feel better as you run

➤ An otherwise unaccountable drop in running performance

➤ Abnormal sleep (either too much or not enough)

➤ Unexplained, increased irritability

➤ Frequent minor colds and infections

Training Tip
If your enthusiasm for running is lacking, it's usually not because you're overtrained. You probably just need to make more of an effort to add variety to your running. Try running in different locations, at different times of the day, faster or slower than usual, with a new training partner, and so on.

The more of these symptoms you have had for at least a week straight, the more likely it is that you're overtrained. If so, cut your running by half and limit yourself to a very easy pace.

Good records in your training log will help you note trends in your running. You can get a better sense of if you're on the verge of overtraining, as well as learn how much is too much from past mistakes.

Two things are important to note here about overtraining. How much running it takes to make you overtrained depends on not only how much you've been running lately, but what else has been going on in your life. If there has recently been a lot of stress in your life, even if it's a lot of good stress, your usual running routine is going to take more out of you. Be more careful about not overdoing it when you're deep in the weeds of a major project at work, or you've just moved, or a loved one is ill in the hospital.

Also, variation in how you feel from day to day is unavoidable in running. So any of those signs of overtraining might hit you on a given day. Don't immediately assume that you're on the verge of falling apart. It's when a majority of them occur day after day that you're probably overtrained, not just when you're feeling a little sluggish. With more running experience, you'll be better able to know which warning signs are serious, and which ones are transitory and par for the course.

The Least You Need to Know

➤ Setting short-term goals to reach in the next few months keeps you motivated and focuses your running.

➤ Goals should be specific and challenging, but reachable.

➤ A detailed training log of important aspects of your running will help you progress toward your goals.

➤ Running with others of similar ability is one of the best ways to stay motivated.

➤ Avoid overtraining. It can lead to physical staleness, a lack of enthusiasm for running, and injury.

Part 2
The Right Stuff

Running is a low-tech, low-hassle sport. You don't need special skis, or just the right type of wheel for your bike, or a different golf club for every hole. What you do need are good running shoes. They're the most important purchase you're going to make as a runner. You don't have to pay a ton for a good pair—about $70 to $80. But you do need to get a pair that fits your needs. In this part, you're going to uncover the right way to buy a good running shoe and find out what apparel and gadgets out there might make your running easier.

Chapter 7

Sole Mates: Finding the Right Running Shoes

In This Chapter

➤ Why you need good running shoes

➤ The three types of running shoes

➤ Finding the right shoe for you

➤ The best places to buy running shoes

Your most important purchase as a runner is the right shoe. Well, that and the left shoe. What I mean is that running is a simple sport. That's one of my favorite things about it. You don't need to buy a bunch of fancy equipment or fill out forms to become a member somewhere or coordinate court times with others. If you want, it can be as simple as just you and the roads.

But you do need good shoes—and not just any shoes, but good running shoes. When you run, your body absorbs a force of about three times your body weight every time you hit the ground. The right shoes will protect you from all the pounding. This protection will help to keep you from getting injured, and staying injury-free is key to enjoying your running. In this chapter, I'll show you what goes into a good running shoe, how to know which one is right for you, and where to buy them.

Why Running Shoes?

All sports have shoes made just for them, running included. But you'll often see beginning runners hitting the roads in any old shoe they have sitting around in the closet. Tennis shoes, boat shoes, basketball shoes—you name it, people think that they're OK to run in. That's too bad, because those people are probably going to hurt more than they should and not enjoy their running as much. Just as you wouldn't expect to shoot hoops well if you hit the basketball court in bowling shoes, you shouldn't expect to run well unless you're wearing running shoes.

Rules of the Road

If you really want to look like a runner, wear an old pair of running shoes for casual wear. They're a lot more comfortable than most street shoes. Just be sure not to walk around in them if they're too beat up.

What makes a shoe a running shoe? It's made for one thing, moving forward. After all, that's what you want to be doing as you make your way down the road. Unlike, say, a basketball shoe, a running shoe doesn't need to protect your ankles from side-to-side motion, nor does it need to help you jump. It just needs to help your body deal with the repetitive stress of putting one foot in front of the other, thousands of times per mile. So let me say this as clearly as possible: If you're going to run, get running shoes. Your body will thank you.

Footnotes

Not all runners think that shoes are essential. Ethiopia's Abebe Bikila set a world record when he won the 1960 Olympic Marathon. He did so running barefoot over the cobblestone streets of Rome. When he won the 1964 Olympic Marathon, however, he wore shoes.

The Last Shall Be First: Shoe Construction

Running shoes vary greatly from one to another, but all good ones have these basics of construction in common (refer to the following figures):

➤ Outsole, the bottom of the shoe that hits the ground

➤ Midsole, the soft, cushioned part directly above the outsole

➤ Insole, the usually removable part on which your feet rest

➤ Upper, the top part of the shoe that holds the laces

➤ Heel counter, the sturdy back part of the shoe

How these parts of a shoe are built and shaped is what makes one shoe good for you and another one not.

The outsole of a running shoe.

The midsole of a running shoe.

*The insole of a
running shoe.*

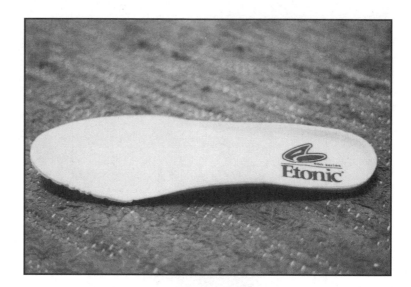

*The upper of a
running shoe.*

The heel counter of a running shoe.

Footnotes

Those ubiquitous Nike waffle soles are aptly named. In the early '70s, when the company was just starting, cofounder Bill Bowerman wanted a way to increase the shoes' traction. So he poured some raw shoe material into the family waffle iron and produced the studded sole that has become standard on most running shoes.

In addition to the midsole, most modern shoes also provide cushioning through technologies that the various running-shoe companies have devised in their labs. The best known is Nike's Air® cushioning. (It's so well known, in fact, that if you ask runners what shoe they wear, they'll often say, "Nike Air," rather than accurately name the model.) Other examples are Asics's Gel®, Brooks's HydroFlow®, and Etonic's StableAir®.

Although the running-shoe companies would vehemently deny it, most of these cushioning technologies are roughly equivalent for most runners. They all do a good job of increasing the amount of shock that the shoe absorbs and therefore decreasing the amount of shock your legs absorb. Some shoes have these cushioning technologies only in the heel, some have them only in the forefoot, and some have them throughout the shoe.

The other major construction part of a shoe is its last. Running geeks love to bandy about this term because it can be used in two ways, so it can confuse outsiders. For the purposes of this book, the last is how the shoe's upper is attached to its midsole. There are three basic types of last:

➤ Board lasting, in which the upper material is glued to a shoe-length board (usually made of paper fiber), and then attached to the midsole

Training Tip
Few things are more irritating during a run than having your shoe laces come undone. Double-knot your shoes before every run. Tie the knots snugly so that the shoe stays firmly in place during your run, but not so tight that you feel pressure across the top of your foot.

➤ Slip lasting, in which, as in a moccasin, the upper material is stitched directly to the midsole

➤ Combination lasting, in which the upper material in the forefoot is attached directly to the midsole, as in slip lasting, while the upper material in the rear of the foot is attached to a board, as in board lasting

You can tell which kind of last a shoe has by removing the insole. Once it's out, you'll see either a solid piece of material (a board-lasted shoe), a piece of material that runs to the arch area (a combination-lasted shoe), or stitches (a slip-lasted shoe). The best last for your shoe depends on how you run, as explained later in this chapter.

The term last can also refer to the shape of the shoe. To avoid confusion, this book uses the term shape. There are three types of shoe shapes:

➤ Straight, in which the shoe is built straight along the arch

➤ Semi-straight, in which the shoe is built so that the forefoot points slightly toward the heel

➤ Curved, in which the shoe is built so that the arch area appears partly carved out

A shoe's shape is best determined by looking at it along the outsole. As with a shoe's last, which shape your shoe should have depends on how you run.

A final piece of construction lingo you may run across while shoe shopping is *dual-density midsole*. In many shoes, you'll see that the inside of the midsole will be darker than the rest. (It's usually gray.) If you push on this area, you'll notice that it's harder than the rest of the midsole. That darker, firmer area is a medial post, designed to add stability to the shoe. Shoes that have a medial post have a dual-density midsole, which means that part of the midsole is denser than the rest.

Track Talk
How your body parts work together as you move is *biomechanics*.
Knowing the biomechanics of your feet and lower legs as you run is key to knowing which running shoe to wear.

The Myth of the Perfect Running Shoe

Buying a running shoe is like buying a computer: There's no accurate answer to the question, "Which one is best?" The right question is, "Which one is best for me?" Like computer users, runners have different needs. I weigh less than 130 pounds and land with the greatest amount of force on my forefeet. That means I need a different kind of shoe than a heavier runner who lands with the most force in the heel, just like someone who does graphic design has different computer needs than an accountant.

All Feet Aren't Created Equal

The best running shoe is the one that best suits how your body, especially your feet, adapts to the stress of running. You want a shoe that best complements how you move through the gait cycle (what running geeks call *biomechanics*).

Running shoes are constructed to address what happens when your feet hit the ground. Ideally, your foot lands on the outside heel, rolls in until your heel is aligned under your lower leg, then becomes rigid as it propels you forward. About half of all runners are blessed with something close to this kind of biomechanics. But many runners' feet roll in too far or continue to roll in as the foot prepares to push off; this type of footstrike is called *overpronation*. And a small minority of runners' feet don't roll in enough; this type of footstrike is called *supination*. The following figures illustrate these three types of running biomechanics.

Track Talk
Overpronation is when your feet roll in too far after they've hit the ground. If you overpronate but don't run in shoes that control the excessive motion, you'll likely be injured.

Track Talk
Supination is when your feet roll to the outside after they've hit the ground. Less than 10 percent of runners supinate. Those who do need shoes with more-than-average cushioning.

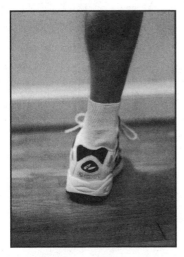

Overpronation (feet rolling in too much).

Neutral stance (feet rolling in about the right amount).

Supination (feet not rolling in enough).

The Three Types of Running Shoes

To address the different biomechanical needs of different runners, shoe companies play with the basics of construction. The shoes that they produce as a result create a continuum of models from heavy, ultrarigid ones to light, flexible ones. There are three main three types of running shoes:

➤ Motion-control shoes, which are designed to combat overpronation

➤ Neutral shoes, which are for runners without significant biomechanical problems

➤ Flexibility shoes, which are designed to provide maximum cushioning for supinators

Although this list is simplifying things a bit, these broad categories are helpful to keep in mind when you start your search for the right running shoe.

Motion-control shoes usually contain these features:

➤ Combination or board lasting

➤ A straight shape

➤ A medial post that extends to the arch

➤ A thick midsole

➤ Heel and forefoot cushioning technologies

Because of these construction features, motion-control shoes are usually the heaviest ones on the market.

Neutral shoes usually contain these features:

➤ Combination or slip lasting

➤ A semi-straight shape

➤ A small medial post

➤ A medium-thickness midsole

➤ Heel cushioning technologies

As you can see, these middle-of-the-road models are designed to suit the majority of runners.

Flexibility shoes usually contain these features:

➤ Slip lasting

➤ A curved shape

➤ No medial post

➤ A thin midsole

➤ Forefoot cushioning technologies

Flexibility shoes are usually among the lightest on the market.

Which Type Should You Wear?

There are many ways to make an educated guess at which type of running shoe is best for you. If you're already running, look at the forefoot of your old shoes. (Don't bother looking at the heel, because almost all runners land on the outside heel. It's what happens after landing that determines your needs.) Neutral runners usually see wear in the center of the forefoot; overpronators often find wear near the big toe; supinators may find wear toward the little toe. Also, examine your old shoes from the back when they're on a level surface. Do the heel counters tilt in significantly? If so, you're probably an overpronator.

Also, if you've had any running injuries, these can give clues as to your biomechanics. Overpronators tend to get injuries caused by soft-tissue fatigue, such as tendinitis and knee problems, because of the extra motion required of their muscles, tendons, and ligaments. In contrast, supinators subject their bodies to great amounts of shock because their feet move through too small a range of motion. As a result, they're susceptible to such injuries as ankle sprains, stress fractures, and shin splints.

If you're new to running, have a friend watch you from behind while you walk and run. Have your friend note what happens to your feet after your heel has landed. If it looks as though the inner part of your heel is still in contact with the ground when you're pushing off to the next stride, then you're probably an overpronator. If your heel appears relatively flat when you push off, you're probably a neutral runner. And if it seems that your foot is moving toward the outside as you push off, you're part of that rare breed of supinators. A good sales clerk at a running shoe store should be able to make the same assessment for you.

Shoe Wear, Tear, and Care

Like everything else in this world, running shoes eventually break down. They just seem to do so much more quickly than other shoes. Remember, with every running step, you create a force of about three times your body weight. Even for the lightest of us, that's a lot to ask our shoes to put up with. So with more miles, your shoes begin to deteriorate. The outsoles get worn out. The midsoles compress. The uppers start to tear. Next thing you know, that shoe that used to feel so good is making your knees ache with every step.

Most runners can comfortably wear their shoes for 500 to 600 miles. In fact, none of the cushioning technologies used in today's shoes are designed to last more than 800 miles. Trying to squeeze more miles than this out of your shoes is the runner's version of being penny wise and pound foolish, because it can lead to injury. In the early '70s, I once wore clean through the outsole of a pair of running shoes; no wonder my calves were killing me at the time! So watch the wear and tear on your shoes. It's a good idea to keep track of how many miles you have on a pair of shoes so that you can better estimate when you need new ones.

Rules of the Road
Your shoes will last longer if you have more than one pair because they won't get broken down as quickly from run to run. Buy two similar, but slightly different, models. Running in different shoes on different days more evenly distributes the pounding on your feet and legs.

Rules of the Road
When your running shoes get wet, stuff them with newspaper or place them in front of a fan. Keep them away from heat, because heat can ruin the midsoles.

Even if you don't meticulously record the mileage on your shoes, always keep an eye on them. If you've worn through a spot in the outsole, ditch 'em. The shoe is so worn down that it's going to throw off your normal stride, and that's a good way to get injured. You should also check the heel counters. If you set your shoes on a level surface and look at them from the back and see that the heel counters point in significantly, they're no longer doing their job of providing support.

After a few hundred miles, you'll probably also start to see wrinkles in the midsole. These wrinkles mean that the midsole is getting compressed and can no longer absorb as much shock as when the shoes were new. When your shoes get in this condition, press a fingernail in the midsole. If doing so leaves a mark that doesn't quickly disappear, it's time for new shoes. Lastly, if you start to notice little aches and pains that you can't attribute to other causes, your worn-down shoes are probably the reason.

There are some things you can do to maximize how long your shoes serve you well. For example, I have a little area on the forefoot of my left shoe that wears down long before the rest of either shoe. I can sometimes get another two or three weeks out of a pair of shoes if I apply Shoe Goo to this spot every two or three days. After I do that, I'm back to normal biomechanically. That is, the wear on my shoes isn't making me run differently; my footstrike is back to how it should be.

You can also extend the life of a shoe by doctoring the inside. I think most of the arch supports and inserts that come with running shoes are weak. As your shoes get a bit worn, you can take out the standard-issue inserts and replace them with a couple of the many commercial inserts available at running shoe stores. Many of these inserts supply extra cushioning, which I find to be helpful as the midsoles of my running shoes compress.

Shopping for Shoes

These days, there are shoes on the market that cost more than the per capita income of some developing nations. Do you really need to spend $150 for a pair of shoes? No doubt, all of the shoes on the market that cost more than $100 are well-made, but that doesn't mean they're necessary. Many running shoes have more to do with marketing hype than with helping you to run better. Let's face it: Like other people, some runners are driven by status. They just have to have the newest shoe with all the fancy colors and the cool logos. If that's you, and if it helps you feel better about yourself as a runner, then by all means, purchase the high-ticket items.

Dollars and Sense

Almost all runners can find shoes that suit their needs for $85 or less. If you're a beginner, I don't think you should spend more than that because you're probably still learning what type of shoe you need. You'll be less likely to be honest about abandoning a model that doesn't work for you if you've just plunked down several days' pay for it.

At the other end of the scale, unless you can find discontinued models on sale, try not to spend less than $60. I know that the dollars can add up fast if you're only getting 400 miles out of a pair of shoes. But shoes that retail for less than $60 are often cheaply made, without enough support and cushioning. They're made in mass quantities out of inferior materials and are dumped on unsuspecting shoppers in megastores. They can lead to injury, and, well, they just don't feel as good as "real" running shoes. Isn't staying injury-free and enjoying your running worth that extra $10 a few times a year?

Rules of the Road
Like car manufacturers, shoe companies like to introduce new models all the time. If you find a shoe that you really like, consider buying more than one pair. If you don't, it might be off the market by the time you're ready for a replacement pair.

The Best Lace Places

The best place to buy running shoes is in a specialty running shop. This is especially the case if you're not sure which shoes to buy. Sure, you'll find a decent selection of shoes in sporting goods stores and even department stores, but those stores lack the knowledgeable salespeople who can help you find the model that's best for you. The workers in a running store are going to be runners like you, who know how important it is to find just the right shoe and who spend their time fitting only runners, not runners along with basketball, football, soccer, and baseball players.

Also, a running specialty store is likely to stock a wider variety of models. The second-tier running companies, who pretty much concentrate on running shoes and don't have big national promotions budgets, make some of the best shoes out there. But these shoes are often hard to find unless you go to a running store.

At a running store, you'll be encouraged to pick up, examine, and try on several models until you find the right match. If the staff won't let you take a short test run in a shoe you're interested in, or if all their recommendations are for the higher-priced models, take your business elsewhere. Keep the following tips in mind when trying on running shoes:

➤ Try on both shoes—one of your feet is probably bigger than the other.

➤ Try on shoes in the afternoon, evening, or after a workout. Your feet are their largest at these times.

Training Tip
Shoes that have too high a heel can shorten and weaken your calf muscles and Achilles tendons. Using your index finger, measure the back of a shoe from the sole to the top of the midsole. The heel shouldn't be much higher than from the tip of your finger to your first knuckle.

➤ Try on shoes while wearing your running socks and any inserts you plan on wearing.

➤ The shoes should flex where your foot does—in the forefoot, not in the middle of the arch area.

➤ When you stand up, there should be a thumb's width from the end of your longest toe to the front of the shoes.

➤ The shoes should feel comfortable immediately, rather than needing a break-in period.

Once you find a model that works for you, then it's OK to buy it wherever you can find it the cheapest. Several running mail-order businesses sometimes offer significant savings over what you'd pay in a store, but I don't recommend buying shoes through the catalogs unless you've previously used the model you're buying.

For More Information...

Other runners are your best source of information on specific models. Runners can get pretty darned opinionated about their shoes, so sometimes you have to take their shoe advice with the proverbial grain of salt. But don't be afraid to ask other runners about which shoes have worked best for them (bearing in mind that they might have different needs than you). If a lot of runners tell you that they don't like a certain shoe, avoid it. Not heeding that advice is like ignoring a group of car owners who all tell you how their transmission went after only 15,000 miles on a certain model.

The two national running magazines, *Runner's World* and *Running Times*, do shoe reviews twice a year in the March and September issues. These reviews coincide with when most new models are released. The reviews do a good job of telling you which of the new models might be right for you.

One note of caution: Although the shoes in these reviews have been tested by the people writing the reviews, the authors usually don't have enough time before their deadlines to run more than 100 miles in any model. As with a car, it's often how a shoe holds up in the long run that determines how happy you are with it. So if you hear rumblings about a shoe from other runners that disagree with what the reviews say, listen to the runners. They'll likely be speaking from past the 100-mile mark.

The Least You Need to Know

➤ Running shoes are the most important purchase a runner makes because good shoes help to prevent injuries.

➤ There's no such thing as the perfect running shoe, only the perfect running shoe for you.

➤ What happens when your feet hit the ground determines which running shoes are best for you.

➤ Expect to pay between $60 and $85 for a good pair of running shoes.

➤ Most runners can get 500 to 600 miles out a pair of shoes before having to buy new ones.

➤ Running specialty shops are the best places to buy running shoes.

Chapter 8

From Top to Bottom: The Right Running Apparel

In This Chapter

➤ How much running apparel you need

➤ The best types of fabrics for running

➤ Staying comfortable while running in the cold

➤ The features of a good sports bra

➤ The best socks for running

My standard outfit for schlepping around the house is an old T-shirt from a race and a pair of jeans. That's true for a lot of runners. You paid for the shirt anyway when you signed up for the race, and wearing it is like donning a scrapbook.

Look around the next time you're in an area with a lot of runners, and you'll notice those shirts being worn for running, too. But more and more these days, you'll see people running in stuff that looks more like what skiers and mountain climbers wear. These days you'll see even the most staid, middle-aged guys running down the street in flashy, multicolor tights.

What's going on here? Do you really need all these different types of clothes to be a runner? In this chapter, I'll describe what basic clothes I think all runners should have and how to know what to wear for increased comfort.

What Do You Really Need?

As you may have picked up by now, I'm a pretty simple guy when it comes to running. When you have a basic, no-frills approach, it's easier to make running more convenient and something that you can and want to do year round. So if you want a dissertation about the latest fashions in running apparel, you're in the wrong book.

Rules of the Road
T-shirts from old races are the runner's unofficial uniform, but be careful what you wear when: It's an unstated, but universal rule that a real runner never wears the shirt from a race in that year's event. You'll look a lot cooler if you have on the shirt from the same race of a few years ago, or better yet, some obscure race from years ago.

If I sound a little snippy here, it's because too many runners are led to believe that they need a different outfit for every five-degree change in weather. Oddly enough, it's usually the apparel manufacturers who will tell you this. One of the big running companies tells its apparel sales crew that there's no such thing as bad weather, just bad apparel. Well, I've run through New England winters for the last 30 years, and trust me, there is such a thing as bad weather.

So despite what the apparel makers and their minions would have you think, you don't need all that much gear to run comfortably year round. In addition, bear in mind that you probably already have some clothes that will fit the bill. Also, you don't have to get all of your gear at once, you can buy it as you need it. Good running apparel will last for several years, so consider your purchases an investment in your health and comfort.

Track Talk
A *singlet* is a tank top designed for running. Because singlets are more ventilated, they are better choices than T-shirts. Most serious racers wear singlets in competition even in weather as cold as 40 degrees. *Tights* are snug leggings for running in cold weather that don't restrict your freedom of movement.

If you're going to run comfortably in most parts of the United States throughout the year, you should have the following in your running wardrobe:

➤ A couple of pairs of running shorts

➤ A couple of short-sleeve and a couple of long-sleeve T-shirts

➤ A *singlet*

➤ Either a pair of *tights* and a heavy top made of similar material or a *running suit*

➤ Gloves and a hat that fit snugly

➤ For women, a couple of *sports bras*

➤ A few pairs of running socks

Obviously, the more you have of each item, the less often you have to do laundry. (Or, if you're not the frequent laundering type, the less your home will smell.) More importantly, as you accumulate a nice amount of running apparel, you don't have to worry about whether your gear has dried from your previous run.

The Cost of Comfort

How much is all of this gear going to cost you? Here are some ballpark figures for items you might not have sitting around the house:

➤ Running shorts: $15 to $30 a pair

➤ Singlets: $15 to $25 each

➤ Tights: $40 to $60 a pair

➤ Tops to go with tights: $40 each

➤ Running suits: $100 to $200 for the set

➤ Sports bras: $15 to $30 each

You can easily pay more for any of these items. One company has a top-of-the-line running suit that retails for more than $300. But that's certainly not necessary. The figures that I just gave you are good guides to getting gear that's high-quality and made for vigorous outdoor exercise.

The winter apparel is obviously the priciest of the lot. That's because this apparel is made of special high-tech fabrics, which I'll tell you more about in just a bit. But remember: Most people get by with either a pair of tights and a heavy top made of similar material or a running suit. Eventually you might want to get both, but that's not necessary. Or you could get a pair of tights, a snug top, and eventually add a nice jacket, and you'd be set for pretty much anything old man winter is going to throw at you.

Track Talk

A *running suit* is a pair of pants and a matching jacket that are warm enough for cold weather running but not so heavy that they restrict your form. Some runners prefer them to tights because they are looser and leave more to the imagination than tights do. Running suits are also known as track suits or warm-up suits.

Track Talk

A *sports bra* is a snug-fitting bra made of the same materials as other exercise gear. You might also hear them called jog bras, because Jogbra was the name of the first company to widely produce sports bras, much like people tend to call all copy machines Xerox machines.

If this seems like a lot of money, bear a few things in mind. As I said, it's not as if you have to go out and buy all of this stuff right when you start running. If you start running in the summer, hold off for a few months on the cold-weather gear until you need it. Even with generous estimates, you can buy enough basic gear to run in comfortably throughout the year for less than $300. That's less than a dollar a day for the sake of being more comfortable and therefore enjoying your running more.

Footnotes

The running apparel industry is even more style driven than the running shoe industry. Unlike shoes, running apparel doesn't change that much from year to year in terms of construction. Pretty much the same types of materials are used every year, and what varies is how they look. You can often find top-quality gear for discounted prices at specialty running stores because they want to make way for the next season's lines.

Fashion and Function

A lot of runners think that what I'm saying here only applies to the hard-core, high-mileage runners. "But I only run a few miles a day," they say. "Why do I need special clothes for running?" You'll see them hit the roads in the winter wearing their old cotton sweats and a parka.

Sure, you can run in that stuff. I certainly put in my share of miles in baggy cotton sweats, heavy coats, and long johns 25 and 30 years ago. But even though back then there wasn't a whole lot of other options, I had the sense that there had to be a better way. I've tripped and fallen because of getting caught on my droopy drawers. And this stuff accumulates water and ice like nobody's business. Back then, my gear always seemed heavy and cold.

So now, when there are better options, I don't understand not taking advantage of them. You want to do whatever you can to make your running easier. Why wouldn't you want to be as comfortable as possible when you run? I have a friend who I run with once in a while. In the winter, this guy likes to run without a hat, no matter how cold and wet it is. And remember, I live in New England, where it can get plenty cold and plenty wet. I've been on runs with him where his hair has had icicles forming on it because he was so cold and wet. I guess it's a macho thing for him, but to me it just seems silly. Running can be difficult enough on its own. Do what you can to make it easier.

Training Tip
Get whatever length and type of running shorts you feel most comfortable with. Most runners prefer some kind of split on the side of the shorts to provide greater freedom of movement. Look for shorts that have a decent key pocket on the inside.

At the other end of the weather spectrum, when it's really hot, you might wonder why you should wear a singlet. Nobody says you have to, but more men who used to go shirtless anytime it got above 70 degrees now wear singlets, even when the temperature is in the 90s.

Why? First, nearly all singlets are light in color. This color reflects the sun's rays. Speaking of the sun, singlets provide burn protection. Runners can be as vain as anyone else, and a lot of men used to take pride in their bronzed torsos. But now we know so much more about how exposure to the sun can lead to skin cancer. I think that's why more men are taking a little bit of cover under singlets. And let's face it—some people are too self-conscious about their bodies to parade around town in only a pair of shorts.

Cotton Isn't King: the Best Fabrics for Running

I'm a pretty low-tech guy. Let's just say that you should probably look elsewhere if you need help putting up your page on the World Wide Web. I'm also a creature of habit and convenience. So when I reach into my drawer for something to run in on a moderately warm day, I'm going to pull out a cotton T-shirt from a race. Given that I go to more than 30 races a year, year in and year out, I'm not at risk anytime soon of running out of them. Many races now give out long-sleeve shirts instead of short-sleeve ones, so I'm covered (sorry, another pun) for much more of the year.

Some of my running partners can't believe how much of my running I do in those shirts. They pay for high-tech gear instead of running in the shirts they get for free from signing up for races. What can I say? I'm as behind the times in my shirt selections as I am in my computer programming skills.

What do they have against the classic cotton T-shirt? Same thing that I have against running in cotton sweats. Cotton feels great against your skin—when your skin is dry. But work up a sweat, and cotton absorbs all of that moisture, and your shirt clings to you. If it's cold outside, you start to feel cold. If it's hot, you get hotter, because your sweat just continues to gather on your shirt rather than evaporating and therefore cooling you like it's supposed to.

What's the alternative? Apparel made from fabrics that provide *wicking*, or, as the apparel designers like to say, moisture transport. When it's hot, the apparel moves sweat from your skin to the surface of the garment. There, it evaporates, so you get cooled. You also feel more comfortable because your running clothes aren't clinging to you as much. When it's cold, and you sweat (it does happen), you stay warmer in wicking fabrics because the moisture isn't held against your skin, so your skin doesn't start to feel clammy.

Most high-tech warm weather gear is made of *CoolMax®*. Some companies have their own version of a similar

Track Talk

Wicking is a term used to describe the process of apparel moving moisture from your skin to the surface of the garment. This process keeps you drier and more comfortable during the course of a run. Because cotton absorbs water so easily, it does a horrible job of wicking.

Track Talk

CoolMax® is the running apparel industry standard for a moisture transport fiber. Its four-channel construction creates 20 percent more surface area than regular fibers do, so it quickly wicks moisture away from your skin to keep you dry. CoolMax retains 8 times less moisture than nylon and 14 times less moisture than cotton.

fiber, but the principles behind the construction are the same. Shopping for running shorts and singlets is therefore pretty much a no-brainer, given that nearly all of the companies use the same materials. Go with what you like and what fits you best.

Track Talk
Microfiber is a broad classification of fiber that's used in a variety of running gear. It's usually nylon or polyester fibers, tightly woven so that sweat vapor can escape from the inside while the fiber remains quick-drying and wind- and water-resistant from the outside. Microfiber apparel usually has a soft, silky feel.

Most running shorts these days have a CoolMax liner and some sort of *microfiber* shell or outer part. At first glance, the shell might look like the 100 percent nylon shorts that were standard for running shorts 20 years ago. But feel them, and you'll notice how much more comfortable they are. They do a heck of a lot better job with the elements than the old nylons did.

My brother, Charlie, and my co-author, Scott Douglas, swear by CoolMax T-shirts for running in moderate weather. Some companies make long-sleeve versions, and these are great choices when there's bit of a nip in the air, but it's not so cold that you need to break out the heavy-duty winter gear. You can find short-sleeve CoolMax shirts for about $20, long-sleeve ones for about $5 more.

Winter Wear

I'm not as stuck in my ways when it comes to winter running gear. I've run through enough Boston winters to know that you're only defeating yourself if you skimp on your cold weather apparel. But as I said, getting some basic high-tech gear doesn't have to bankrupt you.

Track Talk
Layering is dressing to run in the cold with a few light layers. Dressing this way keeps you warmer than wearing one layer of heavy clothes because heat is trapped between the layers. Layering also keeps you more comfortable because a few light layers allow greater range of motion, and as you warm up, it's easy to remove a layer.

The key to dressing comfortably for winter running is *layering.* You've probably heard about layering from outdoorsy types. What they mean when they talk about it is the same as what I mean—wearing a few light layers rather than one bulky one as a way to stay warmer and more mobile.

You could pile on three cotton shirts and technically meet the several-light-layers definition, but once you get going on your run, you sure wouldn't be comfortable, for all the reasons I talked about in the previous section. For running, each layer has a purpose, and there are different types of fabrics to meet the different purposes of different layers.

The Base Layer

The layer closest to your skin, the base layer, should wick moisture away from your skin to the next layer. So what you want for this layer is a material that is like CoolMax, but a bit heavier. A well-known example is polypropylene. Most of the apparel companies have special names for their versions of these slightly heavier fabrics, such as Nike Dri-F.I.T.®, Asics Corium®, and Hind DryLete. All of them have the same basic construction. The thin fabric consists of two layers. The one closest to the skin is what the apparel people call hydrophobic, or water-hating. It moves sweat to the top layer of the material, which is what called hydrophilic, or water-loving.

In dry, windless conditions down to the low 40s, many runners feel comfortable with just this base layer on. (It's got to be pretty cold before you need more than one layer on your legs when you're running.) So if that temperature sounds like close to the coldest you'll be running in, you're pretty much set with a pair of tights and a snug top made from one of these microfibers.

Running Suits

Sometimes you want a layer on top of your base layer. This is where running suits often come into play. These suits act as an outer shell to keep out wind, snow, and rain while allowing sweat vapor to move from your base layer to the surface. The most famous example of an outer layer fabric is Gore-Tex®. Gore-Tex is pretty bulky for running, however. You can still find running suits made from Gore-Tex, but they're not the most comfortable suits on the market anymore. Newer materials, such as ThinTech and Activent™, do as good a job of keeping wind and water out, but they're lighter and more breathable.

I'm a running suit guy much more than a tights wearer, but that's a matter of personal preference and, like wearing those cotton T-shirts, probably just a habit. If you live where running in the winter is going to mean pretty frequent run-ins with cold precipitation, then I'd go with a suit over the tighter stuff. Under your suit you can wear a pair of shorts and whatever thickness of shirt you need to feel comfortable.

In the nastiest winter weather (I'm thinking of my running friends in Minnesota here), you probably want a third layer between the base and shell layers. This layer is called an insulating layer. You want a top for this layer that's going to be pretty much a duplicate of your base layer so that it will help to keep moisture off of your skin.

Should You Top It Off?

When to wear a hat, like so many apparel choices, varies from runner to runner. We've all heard that a lot of body heat is lost through your head. To some runners, this fact means that they always want something on their head. But other runners, especially those who produce a lot of heat, know that this fact means that if they wear a hat, then their hair will get wet with sweat. When this happens, your hair can freeze, and you'll be a lot colder than if you didn't have a hat on. For about $25, you can find hats made of materials with wicking qualities to solve this dilemma.

Rules of the Road
If it's cold enough to run in tights, then you should probably have gloves on. That's because when you run in cool weather, more of your blood circulates in the core of your body, so your extremities get colder. Many runners wear gloves even if they're out in only shorts and a long-sleeve T-shirt.

Another good compromise is to wear a band that just covers your ears. This band protects your ears, which can be especially susceptible to frostbite, but it also allows you to blow off a little steam.

The Gloves Controversy

The gloves versus mittens question is also up to you. Mittens trap heat better, but running in them doesn't feel as natural as running in gloves does. But gloves can make your hands feel colder because your fingers are more spread out. Again, it depends how you react to cold. You can find gloves and mittens with wicking qualities for about $15. When the weather is not especially frigid, cotton gardening gloves, which cost only a few dollars, work fine.

Chest Protectors: the Importance of Sports Bras

There's no evidence that running damages breasts. Still, almost all women runners, regardless of breast size, prefer to run in a sports bra. It is a must-have piece of apparel for women runners.

What you wear over your sports bra depends on the weather and your modesty. During the hottest parts of the year, some women have no qualms about heading out for a run with nothing on top but their sports bra. Sports bras aren't revealing like other bras, and you're going to stay more comfortable in the heat the less that you have on. After all, those men you see running without shirts are doing so to stay cooler, not to improve their social lives. Understandably, some women aren't going to feel comfortable being seen like that in public. If that's you, go with a lightweight singlet over your sports bra. A few companies even make combination tops, with the bra built into the singlet.

Footnotes

Two women created the first running bra in the late 1970s by sewing two jockstraps together. This bra was their attempt to come up with a better alternative to what women runners commonly did then—wrapping themselves in ace bandages or wearing a size-too-small bra. The creators of this prototype went on to found the company Jogbra®.

Because your sports bra is going to fit snugly against your skin, you want it to have some wicking properties. Try a cotton/polyester blend. The polyester will move sweat to the surface and will provide more durability than cotton alone. If you need extra support, look for a bra that has Lycra in it as well.

Keep these fitting tips, offered by the American Running & Fitness Association's executive director, Susan Kalish, in mind when choosing a sports bra:

➤ A sports bra shouldn't have exposed seams inside, because these can chafe you.

➤ The shoulder straps should be about 1/2 to 3/4 of an inch wide. Straps that are narrower than that might dig into your shoulders.

➤ Don't buy a sports bra with clasps; these can dig into your skin. Get a sports bra that slips over your head.

➤ The bra should have a wide elastic chest band to keep it from riding up.

➤ Get a bra as close as possible to your usual size. If you can't fit your thumb under the shoulder straps and elastic chest band, it's too small. If a bra slips off your shoulders, it's too large.

Unlike you might do with regular lingerie, don't buy a sports bra off the rack because it's your size. Always try it on before you buy it. In the dressing room, run in place, swing your arms around, and so forth to make sure that it will move with you.

Sifting Through Sock Selections

Given that a few running nuts out there hit the streets without wearing shoes, it shouldn't be too much a surprise to learn that some runners choose to run without socks. You used to see a lot more of it than you do now, in part because that's how Jim Fixx appeared on the cover of his famous book, *The Complete Book of Running*. But most runners have learned that they're probably going to be more comfortable if they run in socks. The inside materials of shoes can chafe unsocked feet during a run. And your running shoes probably smell nasty enough without sweat pouring right into them from otherwise uncovered feet!

There's certainly no lack of socks to choose from. That broad selection is good, because you're going to go through running socks like no other item of running equipment, shoes included. The good news is that you can find high-quality socks for running for just a few dollars a pair, although, as with everything else in running apparel, you can pay three or four times that much if you want top-of-the-line stuff.

Rules of the Road
Your socks will most likely wear out first in the heels and the balls of the feet. When you start noticing little friction blisters in these areas, it's time to get new socks.

I run in pretty basic, low-cut, white socks. As with shoes, the most important features are fit and comfort, not high-tech claims. Socks are usually available in two to four sizes. Make sure you wear the size that fits your foot. Wearing a sock that's too loose or too tight is as bad as wearing a shoe that's the wrong size.

Footnotes

In the 1988 Olympic Marathon, Mark Conover dropped out at 12 miles because his socks had given him bloody blisters. These socks were made of a high-tech, synthetic fiber. Conover should have stuck with his usual socks. Earlier that year, he had won the Olympic Marathon Trials wearing socks from a three-pair-for-$4 bundle from J.C. Penney!

How thick a sock you run in depends on what's most comfortable to you. Some runners like extremely thin socks because they like to feel the road when they run. (These are probably the people who used to run without socks.) On race day, especially, many runners want as little sock as possible. But sometimes, socks that are too thin will slip around inside a shoe. This can lead to blisters and can detract from a shoe's stability.

Other runners are from the more-is-better school and like a thicker sock because it provides more cushioning. But if your socks are too thick, they can make your shoes too tight and inhibit your normal biomechanics. Runners who have more than one pair of shoes will sometimes wear different thicknesses of socks with different shoes. This strategy makes sense, given the importance of a sock fitting just right within a shoe.

You might see socks specially marketed as running socks. What this usually means is that the socks have extra padding across the ball of the foot, toes, and especially in the heel area. This extra padding cuts down on shock and protects important areas that can blister. There's also usually padding or a tighter area through the arch to allow the shoe to fit more closely and add better arch support. Some runners don't like this feature because they think it feels too constraining. Again, you should go with what feels best to you.

Training Tip

No matter how minimalist you are about your socks, make sure that they come up higher than the top of the back of your running shoes. Otherwise, they'll slip down during your run and cause friction hot spots on the back of your heel.

As with other pieces of running apparel, socks come in many other fabrics beyond the old standby cotton. Cotton is a fine choice for colder weather running—it's very comfortable, and you probably won't be sweating so much that the sock will absorb much moisture. But when it's warmer, cotton can cause problems. Once the cotton fibers become saturated with moisture, the socks might bunch up inside your shoes and cause blisters. It's just not a whole lot of fun to be running down the road on a hot day and feel your wet feet squishing around in your shoes.

Socks made of synthetic fibers are usually better about wicking moisture away from your skin. The most commonly used synthetic fibers in running socks are acrylic, polypropylene, and CoolMax. Sometimes these fibers are blended with cotton, and sometimes they'll make up the whole sock. Polypropylene and CoolMax socks work well year-round. In the heat, they keep your feet drier, and when it's cold, they keep your feet warmer by keeping moisture away from the skin. But these socks are more expensive than cotton or acrylic blends and often aren't as durable. That's especially true if you ignore the instructions that come with these high-tech socks and throw them in the laundry with your old cotton tube socks.

How long your sock should be is completely up to you. You don't often see runners in over-the-calf socks anymore because these can feel as though they're inhibiting your motion. But as for the other main options—roll-down, quarter-length, or crew—go with whatever works best for you. You might want to go with a slightly longer sock in colder weather just so you can be sure that your pants or tights more than cover the top of them.

The Least You Need to Know

➤ You can buy enough apparel to run in comfortably year-round (shorts, shirts, and cold-weather gear) for less than $300 total.

➤ In moderate weather, cotton clothes are fine to run in, but in hotter or colder weather, they can be uncomfortable once they get wet.

➤ For the greatest comfort in hot and cold weather, run in clothes that have wicking qualities, which is the capability to move moisture from your skin to the garment's surface.

➤ CoolMax is the industry standard for a wicking material in running apparel.

➤ The key to staying comfortable during winter running is to dress in layers.

➤ A good sports bra should fit snugly and have wicking qualities.

➤ The most important features of running socks are fit and comfort, not the type of fabric they're made of.

Gadgets on the Go

In This Chapter

➤ What running watches and digital chronometers can do for you

➤ How to use a heart rate monitor

➤ What to know before you buy a treadmill

One of the things I like most about running is that it's so low-tech, and I'm not just saying this because I still haven't figured out how to program my VCR. I like how elemental running is—usually, it's just you, a decent pair of shoes, and Mother Nature. That part of running is never going to change—running down a dirt road on a lovely spring day is pretty much the same today as it was 30 years ago.

In those 30 years, however, a lot of new gadgets have been introduced that are supposed to make running better. I don't like most of them. They just get in the way of the basic act of getting out the door and moving under your own power. In fact, I suspect that one of the reasons for running's growing popularity is that it acts as an escape from the overly digitized world. That said, there are a few gizmos that I think can be helpful to many runners. In various ways, running watches, heart rate monitors, and treadmills are gadgets that can add to the enjoyment of your running by making it more convenient and productive. If only I could say the same for my VCR.

Watch It

Soon after President Clinton took office, the *Washington Post* did a story on how horrible it was that the leader of the free world was meeting foreign dignitaries wearing a $45 hunk of black plastic instead of an elegant Rolex. Whoever wrote that story obviously isn't a runner. If the author had been, he or she would have known that President Clinton favors his digital sports watch because it's the single best techno device for runners ever invented.

Marking Time

The best thing about running watches is that they give you freedom. This statement might sound counterintuitive—isn't timing your run going to make you feel more pressured? Not when you do it correctly.

Track Talk

Splits are times en route to a longer distance. For example, most 10K races have markers at every mile along the way so that you can check your mile splits. Knowing your splits is the best way in a race to know if you're running at the right pace to meet your goal.

Training Tip

When you're timing yourself and checking splits in cold weather, wear your watch on the outside of your sleeves or jacket. That way, you can see your running time without having to dig your watch out from beneath layers of clothes.

Yes, many runners use their watches to meticulously record all of their *splits*, that is, their intermediate times en route to a longer distance. That kind of timing can be good, especially when you're doing specific workouts to improve your performance at an upcoming race. When you're doing these kind of workouts, it's sometimes hard not to feel like your entire worth as a runner for the time being is decreed by your watch.

But one of the main ways that I use my watch is on a regular, easy run when I feel like exploring. I love the feeling of freedom that running can give you—you head out your door, and it's completely up to you where to go. If 10 minutes into your run, you feel like taking a detour off of your usual route, well, who's stopping you? When you have a running watch on, you can make that detour and not wonder if you ran farther or shorter than usual. That's because the main feature on these watches is a stopwatch, or chronometer. All you have to do is start the chronometer at the start of your run, go wherever you want, and stop the watch when you stop running.

Say you normally run for half an hour. If you feel like you're running at about the same pace that you usually do, then you most likely are. There's no use in quibbling with yourself about a potential extra tenth of a mile here or there. It'll all even out eventually. This frees you to start your watch, head off in an unfamiliar direction for 15 minutes, turn around and run home.

The chronometer feature is especially useful when you're traveling and have to run in completely alien territory.

When I'm in a new place, I start my watch, run at my normal training pace for however long I want, and rest assured that I've gone about as far as I would at home. Using your watch this way is also a good way to make new courses at home. Say you have a loop through your neighborhood that you're calling a three-miler. See roughly what your average time is for that loop over the course of several runs, and then chart out other courses that you can run in that time. These new courses will be about the same length as the neighborhood loop.

Things That Go Beep in the Night

If the only feature you used on your running watch were the chronometer, it still would be useful. These days, however, the good running watches have more sophisticated features built into them that can help you in other ways. One feature that a lot of racers use is the lap counter. Don't let the name fool you—it's not designed to be used only on the track. You can use it anytime you want to check and record your splits en route to the finish of a run.

Say you're running in your local Fourth of July five-mile race. You start your watch when the race begins. When you pass the one-mile mark, you hit the lap feature. The watch records the intermediate time. At the two-mile mark, you do the same thing. Again, the watch records your intermediate time. Most of the good watches will then show the elapsed time since the last time you hit the lap feature and so on at every mile marker until the finish.

Training Tip
Don't time every one of your runs. When you know that you're going to run one of your regular routes, and you're just planning on running easy, you don't need to time yourself. It's very easy to become a slave to your stopwatch. This can lead to overtraining and detract from the fun of running.

Footnotes

Accurate splits were so important to the great Finnish runner Paavo Nurmi that he set world records and won Olympic gold medals in the 1920s while holding a stopwatch in the palm of one hand.

This feature is useful for two reasons. Many of us aren't geniuses when it comes to quick calculation, especially when we're trying to concentrate on running fast. The lap feature does the calculating for you. Say you passed the one-mile mark in 8:30. You hit the lap feature and carry on to the two-mile mark, where you hit the lap feature again. Immediately, the watch lets you know that your two-mile split of 17:10 means that it took you 8:40 to cover the second mile. Uh oh—you were hoping to run 8:30 miles the whole way.

You gradually pick up the pace, and at the three-mile mark, you see that you ran your last mile in 8:20. You relax a bit and run 8:30s for the last two miles and meet your goal.

After the race, you can retrieve your splits from your watch and write them in your training log. This type of recording is a good way to analyze your running to see how you might do better. For example, if your splits show that your first mile is always 20 seconds faster than the rest, and your last mile is your slowest, then you know that you're starting your races too quickly and could improve your overall time if you pace yourself better. Or your splits might show that your middle miles are your slowest, so you need to work more on concentrating hard in the middle of a race, when it seems that the finish line is an eternity away.

Footnotes

What did runners who didn't like holding stopwatches during a race do before digital chronometers were invented? Many would wear a regular watch and hold the hands at noon until the race started so that they could easily calculate their time en route.

Harder! Faster! Slower!

The other feature that runners use most often is the countdown timer. You program the watch to count down a certain time, at the end of which it beeps for a few seconds, and then it starts counting down again until it beeps, and so on until you make it stop. Runners will use this feature if they want to alternate bouts of hard and easy running. For example, you may start your countdown timer and run hard. After two minutes, the timer beeps, which is your signal to run very slowly. Two minutes later, it beeps again, and you start running hard, repeating the process as often as you want.

Yes, it's easy to feel like a Pavlovian dog when you use this feature, but it is very helpful when you're doing faster running of the sort that is detailed in Chapter 19. That's especially the case when you don't have access to a measured surface such as a track, or when it's dark out and you might have a hard time reading your watch. Many runners rely on this "countdown training" to guide them through their hard running in the winter.

Some watches also have a programmable feature that beeps many times a minute. The idea here is that you want to maintain a certain pace and have determined your stride frequency for that pace. You then program the watch so that it beeps to coincide with every time that your right foot should hit the ground while running that pace.

I don't think these beeping pacers are a good idea. There's just too many variables in effect for them to guide you to your desired pace. Your stride length and frequency are going to change during a run or race, depending on how hilly the terrain is and how tired you're feeling. Only when you're running on a track is the surface going to be the same throughout your run, and tracks are so calibrated that you can check your splits often enough to know whether you're hitting your desired pace. Also, I'm a big believer in running how you feel, not how fast a beeping watch tells you to.

You can find a good running watch with a chronometer, lap counter, and countdown timer for about $50 (see the following figure). Get one that's water-resistant so that you can wear it in the rain. If you run in the dark often, look for one with an illuminating backlight that you can easily switch on and that stays lit for a few seconds.

A running watch helps you monitor your progress as a runner.

Heart Rate Monitors

Running, like all aerobic exercise, is all about getting your heart rate up. All of those benefits of running that I told you about in Chapter 2 come when you raise your heart rate above a certain level and then keep it there for at least 20 minutes. In Chapter 3, I showed you good ways to know whether you've reached that range, including the talk test and the perceived effort scale. For most people, those vague guidelines are enough to be able to tell whether they're working hard enough to get the physical benefits of running.

But some people figure that if fitness all stems from what your heart rate is, then why not go right to the source? Why not measure your heart rate (pulse) while you run to make sure that you're at the right intensity? Doing so accurately used to be nearly impossible. Ever try taking your pulse while you're running? You can't get a good count. And if you stop to take your pulse, it quickly drops, so your figures are wrong. Besides, who wants to keep stopping during a run to do math?

105

Enter the heart rate monitor. It enables you to check your heart rate throughout your run without having to stop and do any sort of counting. You just look down at your watch as you would to check the time. Even that isn't necessary with some models. With these models, you program the range of heart rate that you want to run at, and the monitor beeps if you get above or below that range.

The ABCs of Effort

Before looking at heart rate monitors specifically, let's delve a bit further into heart rate in general. There are many good reasons to use your heart rate as the guiding force in your running, but doing so has drawbacks as well.

Training by heart rate is good because if you know what numbers to use, there's no more accurate way to gauge your running. When you head out for a run around your neighborhood, how do you know what your pace is? Even if you compare your splits along the way to what you usually run, who's to say that you know what the earlier times mean? If the terrain is hilly, or the weather is warm, or you've been fighting a cold, or you got a bad night's sleep, your pace from day to day will be affected. Heart-rate training proponents like to point out that heart rate monitors take all of those factors into account, and they do so in a way that helps you to progress in your training with less risk of injury and burnout.

Track Talk
The greatest number of times that your heart can beat in a minute before it plateaus is your *maximal heart rate*. This figure doesn't change as you become more fit; what changes is how hard you have to run to reach it.

The theory is that your heart rate can reach two extremes: your resting heart rate and your *maximal heart rate*. Remember resting heart rate from Chapter 6? It's the lowest number of times that your heart beats in a minute. Generally, your resting heart rate decreases as you become fitter because as your heart becomes stronger, it doesn't have to work as hard to pump the blood that your body needs when you're sitting around or sleeping. The average American has a resting heart rate of 72. Aerobically fit people usually have heart rates of around 60, and some hard-core distance runners have pulses of 40 or lower.

Your maximal heart rate is the highest rate that your heart can reach. Unlike your resting heart rate, it doesn't change as you become fitter. Your maximal heart rate is set at birth. Past the age of 30, it decreases by about one beat each year, although it doesn't decline as rapidly in very fit people. Most beginners should run at about 60 to 70 percent of their maximal heart rate. In that range, you're going fast enough to get the benefits, but not so fast that you're continually out of breath and running so hard that you're more likely to get frustrated or injured. In that range, exercise should feel good.

Your resting heart rate and how hard you have to work to run in the 60 percent to 70 percent range vary from day to day. Heat, hills, stress from work, lingering fatigue from a few bad nights of sleep, dehydration, caffeine—all of these factors can elevate your heart rate. What this means is that if you monitor your training by your running pace, then maintaining that pace is going to be harder from one day to the next. If it's 50 degrees outside and you've spent a restful day with the Sunday paper and you run on a flat course, your nine-minute miles arc going to feel a lot easier than if it's a hot Wednesday, and the office was miserable, and you started your day with three cups of coffee, and you're running a hilly course.

Heart rate monitors allow for these differences. In a sense, your heart doesn't care about all that stuff that happened today at the office. It just wants to be worked at a level of effort that's between 60 percent and 70 percent of its maximum. That's going to mean running slower after that stressful day at the office than on that blissful Sunday. No big deal—you've achieved the same aerobic benefits from both runs.

Probably the biggest benefit of heart rate monitors for most runners is that they can help you to keep from working too hard. Sure, you can use monitors to help you stay above that moderate 70 percent-of-max threshold, and many serious racers use them just for that. But recreational runners can use them for the opposite end to great benefit. Using a heart rate monitor can prevent you from overdoing it so that you can continue to progress in your training. Remember, consistent, moderate running is the key to progressing, not intermittent hard bouts of exercise that leave you frazzled and possibly hurt.

Getting to the Heart of the Matter

OK, so this heart rate training might be for you. But how do you know if and when you're in that magical 60 percent to 70 percent of maximal heart rate that gives aerobic benefits without increased risk of burnout and injury? Here's where heart rate training can get tricky, especially if you don't like the whole idea of quantifying something that can be as free-flowing as running.

If you're going to train between 60 percent and 70 percent of your maximal heart rate, then you need to know what that top figure is. You've probably seen this or that formula for determining your maximal heart rate. The most famous one is 220 minus your age. Say you're 40 years old. This formula would say that your maximal heart rate is 180 (220–40). Using this number, you should run fast enough to get your heart rate up to between 108 (60 percent of 180) and 126 (70 percent). Sounds simple even for an idiot, right?

Unfortunately, any formula that you use to calculate your maximal heart rate is going to be inaccurate. The formulas are based on the average maximal heart rates for a person of a given age. So an average 40-year-old has a maximal heart rate of 180. Trouble is, your maximal heart rate may be as much as 20 beats above or below this average. Remember that maximal heart rate is something you're born with; it isn't a reflection of your fitness.

If you have that base level of fitness and want to find your maximal heart rate, here's how. If you run a 5K race and can honestly say that by the end you were working as hard as you can, then your heart rate at the finish is probably within a few beats of your maximal heart rate. Or try this test: Warm up with some very easy running for 10 minutes or so. Do a few accelerations of 15 to 20 seconds at a pretty fast pace. Catch your breath, and then run as hard as you can for two minutes. Pace yourself so that you maintain about the same speed throughout. If you run as hard as you can, you'll most likely be within two to three beats of your maximal heart rate by the end of the run. If you aren't sure whether you gave an all-out effort, jog for 10 minutes and repeat the test. Some runners find that they get a slightly higher heart rate if they perform this test uphill.

You can do these tests without wearing a heart rate monitor if you take your pulse for six seconds almost immediately upon finishing. But if you wait too long or take your pulse for too long, your heart rate is going to start to fall. So take your pulse for six seconds, and then multiply that number by 10 to get a decent estimate of your maximal heart rate. For example, if at the end of a 5K, your heart beats 17 times in six seconds almost immediately after you've stopped, then call your maximal heart rate 170. Once you've determined your maximal heart rate, the rest is easy. Multiply your maximal heart rate by 60 percent and by 70 percent, memorize those numbers, and be sure that you stay within that range on your normal distance runs.

Im-Pulse Purchases

Almost all heart rate monitors work the same way. You wear a thin plastic chest belt around your torso, just above the top of your rib cage (refer to the following figure). At the same time, you wear a wristwatch receiver. (These receivers can double as a chronometer.) The belt picks up your heart rate and sends that signal to the receiver. There, your current heart rate is displayed.

A heart rate monitor can tell you if you're running at the right intensity.

When you run with a monitor, it's tough not to constantly look down at the receiver to see what the readout is, even when you can sense that you're working at the same level of effort as the last time you checked it. To keep you from having to do this constant checking, many monitors have a feature that enables you to program in a floor and ceiling rate. If you go above or below these rates, the monitor will beep, and you'll know that you're out of the heart rate zone that you want to be in.

For example, if 60 percent of your maximal heart rate is 108, and 70 percent of it is 126, then you could program the monitor to beep when you go below or above this range. Then you would know either to pick up the pace or to slow down. If you're going to buy a heart rate monitor, I think you should get one with this feature. This feature makes you more likely to do your normal run without checking the receiver all the time, and it helps to build that ability to listen to your body instead of always relying on signals from the monitor.

Expect to pay between $100 and $180 for a good heart rate monitor. Each works a little differently, so be sure to read the owner's manual carefully. If you want to read more on heart rate training in general, a good book on the subject is *The Heart Rate Monitor Book* by Sally Edwards, Polar Electronic, 1993.

Terrific Treadmills

In March 1993, a runner I know went to bed one Friday night planning to meet a couple of friends for a long run the next morning. When he woke up, he could barely leave his basement apartment, much less meet his friends—more than two feet of snow had fallen overnight! Being the compulsive sort, this dedicated runner hit the roads anyway and somehow slopped his way around in the blizzard for his daily run. The next day, he did the same. The next day, he had Achilles tendinitis so badly that he was incapacitated for more than a month.

"If only I had a treadmill," he thought. An increasing number of runners have obviously had similar experiences and thoughts, because since the beginning of the decade, more treadmills have been sold than any other piece of home exercise equipment. The big reason? Convenience.

The Fast Lane on the Beltway

It doesn't take a blizzard to spur some runners to hop on a treadmill. Many owners just aren't big fans of heading out in the dark and cold nearly every day for more than a quarter of the year. Treadmills are a great way to stick with your running through the toughest parts of the year. And that can mean summer, too—

Rules of the Road
You get the same aerobic benefits from doing the same workout outside or on a treadmill. Mechanically, though, the two runs are different. Outside, you push off against an unmoving surface; on a treadmill, you keep up with a moving belt. So do some outdoor running to prepare for races if you do most of your mileage on a treadmill.

some runners retreat to treadmills when it's scorching outside, but air-conditioned inside. How bad can it be always to have a nice, cool bottle of water within reach? Busy parents also appreciate treadmills because they solve the child-care question. These runners keep Junior occupied nearby while they hop on the treadmill for their 30 or 40 minutes of running.

Treadmills have long been a favorite of runners returning from or nursing an injury. The belt on most of them is padded, so you're assured a softer, more level surface with surer footing than you would probably find outside. There's also the matter of control. You can have pretty much any kind of workout you want on a good treadmill, all at the touch of a button. You can play with the incline setting to simulate a hilly run, adjust the pace setting to get in some fast running, or just keep the pace constant and see how long you can comfortably keep up.

Notice that I said "pretty much any kind of workout." One of the few types of workouts that you can't have on a treadmill is a visually interesting one. That's the main drawback of treadmills—it can be very difficult not to feel like a gerbil in a cage. No matter how bad the weather, I would prefer to run outside most days. I like looking at my surroundings, encountering Mother Nature, and all that. But that's me. If treadmills help to make your running easier, then I'm all in favor of your using one.

Training Tip

To account for the fact that you're not overcoming wind resistance when you run on a treadmill, set the treadmill's grade at one percent to better equate running at a given pace indoors and outdoors.

Milling About

How do you know if a treadmill is for you? I strongly recommend that you use one frequently before going out and buying one. Who among us doesn't have a piece of home exercise equipment that accumulates dust more than it does usage? If you think regularly using a treadmill might be for you, join a health club for a month. See what it's like to run on a treadmill a few times a week. Be honest with yourself about whether you'll continue to do so after you've put down some pretty serious bucks to have one in your home.

Training Tip

Don't take the readouts on a treadmill's console too literally. The speed is usually displayed accurately, although it's not uncommon for them to be off a bit. The calories burned display almost always overstates things. Stick with the rough figure of 100 calories per mile.

Here are some ways to beat boredom on treadmills:

➤ Watch the TV news or your favorite sitcom. Next thing you know (you hope), half an hour is up.

➤ Listen to motivational music.

➤ Don't stare at the console—the time will pass more slowly if you do.

➤ Break your run into segments of various lengths and paces rather than one long haul at the same pace on the same grade.

➤ Have a friend run "with" you on an adjacent treadmill. Runners of vastly different ability can run side by side on treadmills.

➤ Run in front of a mirror to monitor your form.

➤ Visualize yourself out on your favorite running route. Imagine where you would be on that route 10 minutes into your run, 20 minutes into your run, and so on.

Also, if you have a treadmill at home, put inspirational posters or pictures nearby. Just do something so that you're not always staring at a wall!

Footnotes

Next time you get bored on a treadmill after 10 minutes, consider this: In his training before he won a 54-mile race in 1994, Alberto Salazar regularly did runs of 35 to 40 miles on the treadmill in his home.

If you have a treadmill in your home, don't stick it in that musty corner of your basement. You're just not going to be motivated to get on it a lot that way. Create as pleasant a setting as you can. Ann Trason, who has the women's world record for 100K (that's 62.1 miles!), has her treadmill near a window that overlooks a grassy hill.

Rules of the Road
Don't work so hard and get so tired on a treadmill that you lose control. One false move, and you could be thrown right off the back.

Also, putting the treadmill near a window gives you the chance to breathe some fresh air during your run, so at least you're not foregoing all the benefits of running outdoors. If you can't be near a window, try to have a fan nearby to keep the air circulating. You're probably going to sweat more on a treadmill because there's not the wind resistance that you encounter outside. So keep a towel handy.

Making the Grade

You've determined that having a treadmill in your home will improve your running by making it more convenient. What do you need to know before you buy one?

First off, you better have a nice bit of disposable income if you want to buy one that's worth the trouble. Although treadmills are available for as little as $400, they're not suitable for regular running. Their belts often stop running smoothly once you put in some miles on them, they're much more likely to break down with regular use, and some of them barely go fast enough to allow you to run with normal form.

Most treadmill devotees say that a good benchmark price is $1,500. Spend that much, and you can be pretty sure that the combination of features and construction will allow you to run smoothly on the treadmill for several years. Of course, there are manufacturers who will be happy to sell you a treadmill for more than twice that much. These high-end models are a little better, but as with buying a car, once you get to a certain level of quality, you start getting diminishing returns for your extra money.

Rules of the Road

Before running on a treadmill, stand on the edge of the belt and get the machine going at a slow walking pace. Then step on the belt and gradually increase the speed to your desired pace.

Because of the expense involved, you should be sure that you're going to use your treadmill regularly before investing in one. If you do decide to go shopping for one, keep these buying tips in mind:

➤ Shop at a store that offers several models, that will deliver and assemble your treadmill, and that provides a maintenance contract.

➤ Take your running gear to the store and run on the model you're interested in for at least 10 minutes. (If the store won't let you, take your business elsewhere.)

➤ Be sure that the treadmill doesn't shake at the top speed that you plan to run on it.

➤ The machine's top speed should be faster than the fastest that you plan to run on it. Same thing for elevation. It's not good to frequently run a treadmill at full power.

➤ You should be able to change the controls easily while you're running without having to alter your form drastically.

➤ The control panel shouldn't shake while you're running.

➤ To keep you from tripping, the belt should start and stop gradually, and the handle-bars should be reachable, but not intrusive.

You also should consider how loud the treadmill is when you're running on it. How much noise is acceptable for you depends on where you'll be using your treadmill and whether others will be near while you're using it.

The Least You Need to Know

➤ The best gadget ever invented for runners is the digital sports watch.

➤ You can find high-quality running watches with all of the features you need for about $50.

➤ Training with a heart rate monitor to determine whether you're running at the right level of effort is the most accurate way to keep from running too hard or too easy.

➤ Running on a treadmill can help you stick with your running by giving you an alternative to uncooperative weather.

➤ Don't buy a treadmill for your home until you've run enough on one elsewhere to be sure that you'll use it regularly.

Part 3
Body Shop

Keep running, and you'll be on more intimate terms with your body than you have ever been. This muscle feels this way, that muscle feels that way. Runners are nothing if not focused on their bodies.

This part is all about making your body the best it can be for your running. You'll learn easy ways to stretch and strengthen some parts of your body in order to make your running easier and prevent injury. You'll also find out about ways to treat injuries, good diets for runners, how other activities can help your running, special things that women runners need to know, and how to run in any weather. I guarantee that by the end of this part of the book, you'll know how to keep your body in top working order for running.

Chapter 10

Stretching: The Truth

In This Chapter

➤ Why all runners should stretch

➤ The right way to stretch

➤ The best times to stretch

➤ Essential stretches for runners

➤ How massage helps runners

This has happened to almost everyone who has run for a while: You're pushing against a wall or car or other big, immovable object, with one leg bending toward the object, the other behind it and straight. Invariably, someone comes along and says, "Need help holding it up?"

Ha, ha. What these people often don't know is that you're doing one of the classic runner stretches, the wall push-up. It might look funny, but it sure does a great job of stretching your Achilles tendons and calves, which can get sore and tight with running.

Track Talk

Flexibility is your ability to move through a full range of motion. Along with aerobic capacity, muscular strength, and muscular endurance, it's one of the key components of fitness. When you're more flexible, running is easier because muscles, ligaments, and tendons don't have to work as hard to maintain a given pace. Maintaining decent flexibility is an important aspect of remaining injury-free.

As you probably know, those aren't the only parts of your body that can get sore and tight from running. In this chapter, I'll show you how to stretch to increase your *flexibility* throughout your body so that you can run with more efficiency and fewer injuries. I'll also let you in on a related secret that has helped to keep me on the road for so many years.

Flexible Flyers: Why Not to Be a Tightwad

Before showing you how to stretch, I want to tell why you should stretch. Some runners never stretch and try to cover up the real reason they don't (laziness) with silly theories. The main reason offered for not stretching is summarized by the supposedly rhetorical question, "You never see a racehorse stretch, do you?" What they're trying to say is thoroughbreds seem to be able to run pretty well just by running. To suggest that humans need to do more to run is to argue with nature.

Yes, it's true that you don't see racehorses stretch. You also don't see racehorses sit behind a desk eight hours a day, or run on asphalt, or start running after being sedentary for the previous 40 years. I don't see racehorses eating spaghetti, either, but that doesn't mean I think that runners shouldn't. So maybe when we're all bred solely to run fast and spend our days trotting around on dirt tracks, we can forego stretching. In the meantime, all runners, at least of the human variety, should stretch.

As running strengthens your muscles, it also shortens and tightens them. This is especially true of the prime movers on your back side: your Achilles tendons, calves, hamstrings, butt, and back muscles. You're will feel better running, as well as most of the rest of the time, if these muscles are limber and can move through a wider range of motion.

Footnotes

Even the best runners in the world need to work on their flexibility. In 1982, Britain's Dave Moorcroft set the world record for the 5K. At the time, he joked that he was so tight that he could barely reach past his knees. But soon after, he began to have chronic leg injuries that put an early end to his career.

By way of analogy, think about in which instance you'd rather launch into a sprint: immediately after having been driving for the past two hours or after having walked around the block? Intuitively, you know that you feel better running when you're looser, no matter what the racehorse fans would have you believe. And just as you're more limber at a specific time if you've been moving around, you're more limber in general if you regularly incorporate stretching into your running program.

Another important reason that all runners should stretch is because properly doing so will lower the risk of injury. Note that I said "properly." I'll get to what that means in a bit. What I want to say here is that the anti-stretchers will often give you anecdotal evidence about runners they know who stretch and still get injured. To that I say, "Yeah, and…?" No one has ever claimed that stretching will prevent injury. And when it's done wrong, it most definitely can cause injury.

But when stretching is done right, it can help keep you injury-free. That's true for the same reason that a short, taut rope is more likely to break under a given amount of force than a longer one of the same strength. In both cases, the shorter, tighter fiber is being asked to do a relatively greater amount of work, and eventually, it will tear from the task. When your muscles and connective tissues are more supple, they can more easily absorb and distribute the repetitive shock that running subjects them to.

Because of these benefits, stretching has some adherents who are as zealous about doing it as some people are opposed to it. I know some runners who couldn't care less about what you think regarding their political positions, but will subject you to hours of debate if you dare question their approach to stretching. You'll see these runners at tracks sometimes, stretching for a good half an hour on the infield, and then jogging a mile and heading home. Some runners, it seems, get so carried away with their stretching that they spend far more time on it than they do putting in the miles.

Footnotes

Some runners are more dedicated to their flexibility work than others. Immediately after winning his second Olympic Marathon in 1964, Abebe Bikila ran to the infield of the track, got on his back, and began a series of limbering exercises!

Now, I'm all for people doing whatever exercises they find make them feel good. But this is a book for runners, not would-be yoga masters. It's hard enough to find time on a regular basis to keep up a consistent running program. I don't want people to think that on top of their running, they need to spend several hours a week stretching. That's not necessary, and I think you're more likely to stick with a stretching routine if it becomes just that, a routine, and an easy one at that.

How much time should you allow for stretching? The program I outline in this chapter should take only about 15 minutes to do. If you can do that four times a week, that's only one hour out of the 168 hours in a week. I don't think that's too much time to spend to contribute significantly to making your running easier, more enjoyable, and less interrupted by injury.

Don't Go Ballistic: The Right Way to Stretch

For many of us, our early memories of stretching come from gym class. There, we did windmills, where we jerked one side of our body toward the other while touching one hand to the opposite foot. We probably also remember stretching being an exercise in group counting, with a leader saying, "One, two, three," and the group responding, "Four!" So even when we weren't bouncing around, we were holding our stretches for a few seconds, at best.

Track Talk
Stretching your muscles with quick, jerky movements is known as *ballistic stretching*. Avoid this method. If you stretch too suddenly and for too short a time, your muscles are likely to become strained, not more limber.

Track Talk
Gradually stretching a muscle to the point where you feel a slight pulling sensation is known as *static stretching*. This is the right way to stretch. Static stretching helps muscles to stay limber.

I hope I don't disillusion you too much when I tell you that what you were taught in school wasn't quite the truth about stretching. (And you thought it was only in sex ed class that you were given misinformation.) Bouncy, jerky movements and stretches that are held for a few seconds aren't the kind of flexibility exercises that are going to help you as a runner. If anything, they'll hurt you; you're better off not stretching at all if you're not going to do it right.

What is the right way to stretch? A good way to understand the right way is to know more about the wrong ways. The bouncy, jerky stretching I just described is called *ballistic stretching*. It's bad because when you make a movement that lengthens a muscle, its initial reaction is to contract. Think about what happens when you briefly extend a coil, and then suddenly let it go. The same quick return to a shorter state happens when you stretch ballistically. This type of stretching increases, rather than lessens, the amount of tension in your muscles. In some cases, it can cause the muscles to tear. That's not a great way to lower your risk of injury.

The right way to stretch is to do so comfortably, gently, and consistently. Improving, or at least maintaining, your flexibility is similar to improving your endurance. As explained in Chapter 3, "Taking Your First Steps," the key to progress in your running is to find a comfortable level of effort and to work out regularly at that level. As you stick with that approach, your endurance will increase, and you can gradually run more, or faster, without any more effort.

The same is true with stretching. Regardless of the specific exercise you're doing, you want to find a point where the muscles you're working on are stretched just enough so that you can feel it, but not so much that it's obvious you're overdoing it. This type of stretching is known as *static stretching*. As with the first part of your running program, when in doubt, ease up. It's better to stretch a muscle a bit less than to overdo it.

As with boosting your endurance, when it comes to flexibility, slow and long are better than fast and short. You should hold all stretches for at least 15 seconds. Thirty seconds is even better. This amount of time encourages increased blood flow to the muscles you're concentrating on, which will gradually elongate them. When you comfortably hold a stretch for 15 to 30 seconds, the muscles will relax. This reduction in muscular tension is what makes you feel looser, both right after the stretch and from day to day when you're consistent with your flexibility program.

After the stretch, relax the muscles you're working on for the same amount of time. Then do the stretch once more, again holding it for 15 to 30 seconds. By the end of the second time you've done a certain stretch, you'll probably notice that your flexibility in that area is greater than when you began, just like your normal training pace is easier 10 minutes into a run than at the beginning.

Rules of the Road
Do your stretching on a firm, but comfortable, surface. If the surface is too hard, such as a wooden floor, you're not going to be able to relax. If it's too soft, such as a bed, you won't be able to do the stretches properly. A plush carpet is good. You can also find padded stretching mats for about $10.

Some runners find it helps to time their stretches to ensure that they're holding them for that 15 to 30 second range. Many people who say that they can't hold a stretch for that long say so because they hold their breath while they stretch. After 10 or so seconds, they let the stretch go because they need to breathe. You should always be able to breathe normally while stretching.

Scheduling Stretching

In an ideal world, all of my runs would go something like this: a gentle warm-up of slow walking and running, lasting about 10 minutes; then 10 to 15 minutes of stretching; my planned run for the day; then 10 to 15 minutes more of stretching. Following this format would mean that when I start the first bout of stretching, the warm-up would have increased blood flow to my muscles, thereby increasing their ability to stretch without injury. That pre-run stretching would also mean I'd start my run less creaky and could more readily feel comfortable at my regular training pace. The post-run stretching would help my muscles and connective tissues maintain their length until it was time to start the whole thing over the next day.

Like I said, that's how things would go in an ideal world, but in reality things are different. I'm not saying that I shouldn't do the routine I've just outlined, just that I don't. I

Training Tip

Do your stretching in a pleasant environment. Many runners like to find a quiet spot where they can relax and focus on their stretching without any distractions. Many runners also like to listen to music while stretching. Listening to a few of your favorite songs is a good way to help pass the 15 or so minutes that you should spend stretching.

Training Tip

If you stretch after you run, change into warm, dry clothes first. Get something to drink and bring it with you to where you'll be stretching. Both of these things will encourage you to spend the time stretching rather than rushing off to the shower or refrigerator.

don't want to be hypocritical here and describe some perfect stretching routine if it's one I know I almost never do. I'm a big believer in keeping running simple. The easier it fits into your busy life, the more that you're likely to stick with it. In terms of stretching, that means hitting upon a routine that you'll do consistently, even if it's not the ideal one.

You can get pretty much everything that you need out of your flexibility program by doing it either before *or* after, rather than before *and* after, your run. So which is better: before or after? If it's going to be one or the other, go with after.

If you limit your stretching to before your run, you won't get as much out of it. First, your muscles are colder and tighter then, so you won't be able to stretch as far comfortably. It's also easier to overstretch then and potentially hurt yourself. There's also a good chance that you'll rush through your routine if you still have your run in front of you; time may be short, and you want to get out the door! All of this is especially true for the many runners who train in the morning before work.

Contrast that with stretching after your run. Your muscles are warm and more receptive to being gently elongated. For this reason, stretching after a run just feels so much better. You're also likely to be more relaxed after your run.

The only times I stretch before a run are when I have a specific sore spot that I'd like to try to loosen up before hitting the road. After races, my calves are usually pretty sore. So the next day, I'll do a few minutes of very gradual work on them before my run. Still, I'll do my regular routine after the run. The only other time that I regularly stretch before running is when I'm going to be running hard. Even then, though, I've usually warmed up with some easy running. At races, for example, I might stretch a bit after getting out of the car, and then do my warm-up of slow running, and then do more stretching before putting on my racing shoes.

Sometimes, you might not have time right after your run to stretch. In those cases, you can still get most of the benefits of stretching by finding a short chunk of time elsewhere in the day. I think you'll make a lot more progress in all areas of your running if you have a flexible (ha!) approach rather than an all-or-nothing outlook.

Say you have a five-mile run planned, but only have time to run three. Getting those three miles in is much better than bagging the whole thing. Same thing with stretching. Stretching after dinner, or while watching TV, or just before you go to bed, might not be ideal, but if that's when you have time for it, doing it then is better than not doing it all because you didn't have time right after your run.

Essential Stretching Exercises for Runners

As I said before, some runners seem to spend more time stretching than they do running. Given that the human body has more than 500 muscles, you could spend all day stretching if you really wanted to work on your flexibility. But you have better things to do than that, right?

What you want to know is which of those more than 500 muscles tend to make your running better. Certainly, you can get more involved than what I'm going to recommend here, but all runners should have a stretch that they do regularly for these areas of the body:

➤ Feet and ankles

➤ Calves and Achilles tendons (the backs of your ankles)

➤ Hamstrings (along the backs of your legs)

➤ *Iliotibial band*

➤ Hips and butt

➤ Groin

➤ Back

> **Rules of the Road**
> To get the most out of your stretching, do your flexibility routine in clothes that won't inhibit your range of motion. Running shorts and a T-shirt are ideal. You want clothes that are loose enough so that you can move through a full range of motion, but not so baggy that they're going to get in the way.

> **Track Talk**
> The *iliotibial band* is a thick, fibrous band of tissue that runs along the outer leg from the hip to the knee. It often becomes tight in runners, especially those who run on slanted surfaces.

You'll notice that these areas are almost all on your back side. Although it feels great and is beneficial to stretch body parts along your front, such as your quadriceps muscles in your thighs, it's the ones along your back side that you have to give the greatest amount of attention.

Everyone has his or her favorite stretches for these various parts. I like to tweak traditional stretches if I can find a way to isolate a body part that I'm having trouble with. So

121

don't think that the exercises I describe are the only ways to stretch theses key body parts. Start with what I explain here, and if you find a way to alter these stretches that works better for your sorest, tightest spots, feel free to experiment.

No matter how closely you follow the routine I outline here, keep these basic guidelines in mind:

➤ Stretch at least four times a week to maintain and improve your flexibility.

➤ Stretch on a flat, firm, comfortable surface.

➤ Stretch in warm, dry clothes that won't restrict your range of motion.

➤ Hold each stretch for 15 to 30 seconds, release it and relax for the same amount of time, and then repeat these two steps.

➤ Breathe normally while stretching.

➤ Stretch only to the point of mild sensation.

With those caveats in mind, let's look at the basic stretches on the following pages that all runners should do some version of.

Feet/Ankle Stretch

As illustrated in the following figure, start the feet/ankle stretch by sitting with one leg flat and straight on the floor; the other leg should be at roughly a 90-degree angle, with your heel on the floor so that the toes of that foot point toward the ceiling. Grab the toes of your bent leg and pull them toward your chest. After 15 seconds, point them as far as you can in the other direction. You should feel the stretch along the top of your foot, where it joins your ankle. Relax your foot, then repeat the stretch in both directions. Switch the position of your legs, and do the stretch twice for the other leg.

The feet/ankle stretch.

Calves/Achilles Tendon Stretch

To stretch your calves and Achilles tendons, stand facing a wall with the palms of your hands flat against the wall and your toes pointing toward the wall, as shown in the following figure. You should be at arm's length from the wall. Place one foot about 10 inches in front of the other. Lean into the wall, bending your forward leg. You should feel the stretch in the calf muscle and Achilles tendon of your back leg. Relax, then repeat the stretch for the same leg. Switch the position of your legs, and do the stretch twice for your other leg.

The calves/Achilles tendon stretch.

Hamstring Stretch

Begin the hamstring stretch by lying on your back, as shown in the following figure. Wrap a towel or rope under the ball of one foot. If your hamstrings are very tight, keep the other foot on the floor with the knee of that leg bent. If you're more flexible, straighten both legs flat on the floor. Slowly raise the foot with the towel around it toward the ceiling. Don't use the towel or rope to pull your leg down; instead, push your foot up. Straighten the leg being stretched only as far as feels comfortable. You should feel the stretch along the back of your raised leg. Relax, and then repeat the stretch for the same leg. Switch the position of your legs, and do the stretch twice for your other leg.

The hamstring stretch.

Iliotibial Band Stretch

To begin the iliotibial band stretch, sit with one leg bent at roughly a 90-degree angle, as shown in the following figure. Keep the other leg straight and flat on the floor. Place the foot of the bent leg just over the outside knee of your straight leg. Place the elbow of your opposing arm on the outside knee of your bent leg. Push the knee of your bent leg toward your opposing shoulder. You should feel the stretch along the outside of your bent leg, anywhere from the hip to the knee. Relax, then repeat the stretch for the same leg. Switch the position of your legs, and do the stretch twice for your other leg.

The iliotibial band stretch.

Hips/Butt Stretch

Lie flat on your back to begin the hips/butt stretch. Draw one leg toward the other at a 90-degree angle with your opposing arm. Gradually pull your bent leg across your straight leg, as shown in the following figure. You should feel the stretch in your hips and deep in your butt. Relax, then repeat the stretch for the same leg. Switch the position of your legs, and do the stretch twice for your other leg.

The hips/butt stretch.

Groin Stretch

To stretch the groin area, sit with the soles of your feet against each other. Place your elbows against the insides of your knees. Gradually push your legs down so that the outsides of your knees approach the floor. You should feel the stretch on the upper insides of your thighs. Relax, then repeat the stretch.

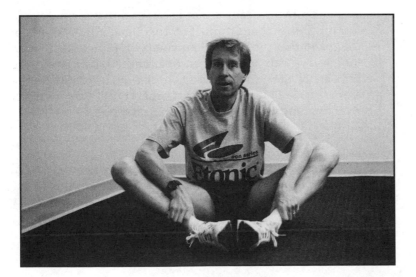

The groin stretch.

Back Stretch

Kneel on the floor with your knees at a 90-degree angle to begin the back stretch. Your back should be flat and your arms locked, with your palms flat on the floor. Simultaneously tighten your abdominal muscles and tilt your pelvis toward your head so that your back arches like that of a stretching cat, as illustrated in the figure. You should feel the stretch from the top of your butt through your lower back. Relax, then repeat the stretch.

The back stretch.

Rubbed the Right Way: Massage

Track Talk

Sports massage involves deep, vigorous work on the main muscle tissues that you use when working out. It's done to loosen overused muscles and to help them release waste products. It's a lot different from the general relaxation technique that most people associate with massage.

You've probably heard stories about cars that seem to last forever, those sedans from 1965 that have 250,000 miles on them and that run better than your year-old model. Those long-lasting cars aren't flukes. Behind their long, healthy lives are owners who regularly check fluid levels, rotate tires, and are equally fastidious about other routine maintenance work that most of us ignore until it's too late.

There are many reasons why I've been able to run for so long, race so much, and seldom get injured: good genes, consistency in my training, and knowing when to back off. But one of the major factors in my longevity is one of the most underrated and is the secret I alluded to in the intro to this chapter. Since 1980, I've been getting an hour-long massage once a week. And the massage is not just any old massage, but a *sports massage*.

I'm including massage in this chapter because it has many of the same benefits as stretching. As with stretching, massage increases blood flow to muscles. This increased blood flow helps to repair the tiny tears, called microtraumas, that occur any time you run or do other strenuous activities. These tiny tears are patched in your muscles with scar tissue; if enough scar tissue accumulates, your flexibility is decreased. Massage helps here because its deep, rhythmic stroking helps to align scar tissue along muscles, rather than across them. This alignment helps to keep you more limber, just like a good stretching program does.

I can hear you already, saying that this is all fine and good for me, but that you can neither afford a weekly massage, nor have the incentive that I do to be so regular with them. It's not my place to tell you what to do with your money, but I flat out disagree with the second point. We're talking the enjoyment of your running here. That's as important for you as it is for me as it is for the fastest people in the world. How are you going to put a financial value on consistently feeling better in your running?

An hour-long massage costs about $40. If this is too much to afford every week, how about every other week? To get any real benefits, you should go at least once a month. Anything less is like starting from scratch, like the guy who checks the oil in his car once a year.

The greatest benefits from massage, as with stretching, come from doing it regularly, even when your body feels fine. Certainly, both can help you when you have an acute problem. But you probably know what I'm going to say next: A good way to avoid getting those acute problems in the first place is to be consistent in your flexibility program, which should include massage.

The two best ways to find a good massage therapist are to ask other runners and to contact the American Massage Therapy Association (AMTA). Try asking other runners first. It's important to find someone who regularly works on athletes and understands that you're there for specific, performance-related reasons, not just to feel better by having those knots taken out of your neck and shoulders. Not that the latter doesn't feel great, but the therapist should spend most of your time together working where you need it—your legs.

Rules of the Road

For sports massage to be effective, you should be able to feel that the therapist is digging deeply into the area being worked on. But that doesn't mean the massage should hurt. Acute pain during a session means the massage is too vigorous. If you're sore the next day, the massage has done you more harm than good.

Footnotes

You can call the AMTA at (847) 864-0123 to find therapists in your area. Be sure to ask about therapists who work with athletes. You'll find some who have the letters "CSMT" attached to their name, which stands for "certified sports massage therapist." Try these therapists first if you can't get a recommendation from a runner. No matter who you wind up calling, find out their experience in working with athletes.

Once you start getting massages, only stay with the therapist if he or she is willing to work with you. I've been with my current therapist for more than five years now. That's because she listens to what I say about where I need work done, rather than just plowing through the same routine, regardless of who is on her table. A good therapist will cater the massage to where you need it most and will remember your body's idiosyncrasies. When you're comfortable with each other and sense that the person you're seeing is catering to your situation, you're going to get more out of the experience.

The Least You Need to Know

➤ A good flexibility program will increase your enjoyment of running and lower your risk of injury.

➤ You can contribute significantly to your flexibility with just four 15-minute stretching sessions per week.

➤ The best way to stretch is slowly and gently, holding each stretch for 15 to 30 seconds.

➤ The best time to stretch is right after you run.

➤ The most important areas for you to stretch are on your back side, especially your calves, hamstrings, butt, and back.

Chapter 11

Pumped Up: Strength Training for Runners

In This Chapter

➤ Why all runners should do some form of strengthening work

➤ Why strength training doesn't mean gaining unwanted weight

➤ Essential strengthening exercises for runners

➤ How to detect and correct muscle imbalances

I'm 5'9" and weigh about 130 pounds. Based on that, you might be as ready to take advice from me on how to get stronger as you would from Elizabeth Taylor on how to build a lasting marriage. I don't pretend to know everything there is to know about lifting weights, but I don't need to. What I know, and what you should care about, is what few simple exercises to do a few times a week to run easier and more smoothly. That's a lot different than what Arnold Schwarzenegger would probably have you doing, but when was the last time he won the Boston Marathon? In this chapter, I'll show you why and how all runners should do some form of strengthening work, as well as some special leg-strengthening exercises that some runners should do.

Ever Notice That Runners Are Skinny?

Before getting down to business, I want to set a few things straight. And no, I'm not just doing this because I'm tired of having sand kicked in my face. Look at pictures of top runners at any distance from the mile on up, and you'll notice one common trait—they're all really skinny! Especially in the arms and torso, these are bodies that make people think more about prison camps than peak health. This impression is particularly prevalent with male runners, in part because our society still equates masculinity with brute strength.

Footnotes

Not all top-class runners fit the 98-pound weakling stereotype. Jim Hage, of Lanham, MD, is a 2:15 marathoner and has ranked as high as eighth in the United States in the marathon. He can bench-press 220 pounds, which is one and a half times his weight. The equivalent for a typical pro football lineman would be bench-pressing 450 pounds!

But appearances can be deceiving. Yes, it's true that in comparative studies, distance runners usually score below average in tests of *muscular strength*, as measured by a one-repetition maximum. But that's largely because of the fact that their weight is also below average. When the figures are adjusted to take into account strength for body size, runners have average strength.

Track Talk
Technically, *muscular strength* refers to how much force you can generate doing one all-out repetition of a given exercise. This quality is important for runners, but not as much as is muscular endurance, the ability to maintain a lower level of work for a long time.

I'm making this point because some people, mostly men, are turned off by running because of how skinny top runners are. Given how we're conditioned to think that bigger is always better, that's understandable, but it's also unfounded. Top runners are born with a body type that predisposes them to thinness, especially when they run upwards of 15 miles a day.

For most people, looking like that is just never going to happen, especially given that almost nobody is going to put in the number of miles that top runners do day after day, week after week. So don't let the looks of a few genetic freaks—I'm including myself here—discourage you from running. You're probably going to lose some weight as a result of your running, and I assume that most of you see that result as good. What you're not going to lose is relative strength.

Hurry Up and Weight

So if running isn't going to make you so weak that you need help bringing in the Sunday paper, then why am I saying that all runners should do some strengthening work? For starters, because everyone should, in the same way that everyone should do some sort of regular aerobic exercise. The American College of Sports Medicine recommends that all adults do two or three *resistance training* sessions per week to maintain and build muscular strength. This recommendation makes sense to me. Being cardiovascularly fit, as you will become through running, is certainly the most important aspect of being fit, but it's not the only one.

More specifically for runners, you'll be able to progress more in your running if you include some basic strengthening exercises in your program. Remember what I said about running form in Chapter 3: You run best when your whole body moves in sync. This type of movement means, among other things, that your upper body flows right along with your legs, rather than being somewhat awkwardly perched atop your legs, contradicting their every move. When you have a basic level of strength in your upper body, you can hold yourself better and more upright as you run. This ability will make a given pace feel easier.

Track Talk
Resistance training involves working a muscle or muscles against force. Common examples include lifting free weights, using an exercise machine, or using your own body to provide the resistance, such as doing push-ups.

Only the Strong Finish First

Decent upper-body strength especially helps you when you tire on a run. For an extreme demonstration of this principle, go watch a race sometime. At the finish, you'll see that the top finishers, no matter how hard they might be straining and striving, are running pretty smoothly. Their shoulders aren't hunched over or somewhere up around their ears; instead, their shoulders are low, and their arms are driving in sync with their legs. Even when they're very tired, one of the reasons that they can keep running fast is because their upper body is strong enough to keep up with their legs.

Then watch for the finishers farther back. Many of them are tired in the arms, shoulders, and back, and you can see it in their form, which has disintegrated greatly from how it was at the beginning of the race. That's partly because they're not as strong relative to the top finishers, no matter how scrawny the first few people across the line might look.

Top and Bottom Working Together

In addition to helping you run more smoothly, a strong upper body will help you to avoid injury. Ron Clarke, who set several world records in the 1960s, used to say that a distance runner couldn't be too strong in the middle. What he meant was that when you run, the shock that comes every time that your feet hit the ground is transmitted

131

throughout your body if your midsection is strong. Strong stomach and back muscles absorb some of that shock, rather than confining it to your legs. The result is that your legs have to put up with less impact force and won't get as overloaded with potential wear and tear.

If you doubt this statement, think of trying to run if your body were like an accordion. With every step, you'd send shock from your feet up your legs to your middle, where, if you're like an accordion, you'd then sag over or almost crumple. That's not how to run smoothly or comfortably!

Bulk Quantities?

Unfortunately, a lot of runners don't believe a word of this advice. They like to point out that if a strong upper body were necessary to run well, then certainly you'd develop one through running. They also like to scare people away from trying to get stronger by warning that lifting weights will make you "muscle-bound" and add tons of unwanted bulk. After all, they'll ask, wasn't losing weight one of the main reasons you started running?

Sounds kind of like the reasoning that the anti-stretchers tried to use in the previous chapter. Obviously, you can run without ever even so much as looking at a weight or contemplating a sit-up, but that doesn't mean that you're going to run as well as you can, or that it will feel as good. Chapter 10 pointed out that running can do some contradictory things to your body; for example, it can tighten the very muscles that are most needed for running. That's why you need to stretch. In the same way, running doesn't affect many of the muscles that, when stronger, will help make running easier. That's why you need to strengthen.

As for worrying about piling on pounds of unwanted bulk, don't. Just as most people who run are never going to have to worry about being as thin as I am because of not being genetically predisposed that way, most people are never going to look like a bodybuilder. The top bodybuilders are as suited to their chosen sport as I am to mine; most people can't look that way, no matter how much they lift.

Rules of the Road
Always protect your back when doing strengthening work. Concentrate on maintaining a slight curve in the small of your back and keeping your shoulders aligned with your hips and feet.

More important, the strengthening program I'm going to outline here would make most of them laugh. That's fine. They work to build maximum bulk. What should concern you is doing a minimum to make your running better. What's necessary for that isn't much and certainly doesn't involve any of the kinds of mega weights that bodybuilders throw around.

If you're still opposed to the idea of strengthening exercises because you're running to lose weight, consider the results of a study that was conducted in the Netherlands a few years ago. In the study, people were divided into a solid group and a slender group. Both groups then lifted twice a week for 12 weeks. As expected, the members of the solid group (the football players of the world) had stacked on significant amounts of fat-free mass during the study. That is, they gained weight in the form of muscle. The slender group, however, was as wiry as ever after the 12 weeks, with no real increase in fat-free mass. The researchers concluded that those with slender body types, which includes most runners, lack the genetic predisposition to bulk up.

If that's the case, then why bother with weights? Because the slender group's failure to gain fat-free mass doesn't mean that they didn't benefit from their lifting program. At the end of the 12 weeks, they had increased their strength by 13 percent, and they had 10 percent less body fat than at the beginning of the study. They were stronger and leaner, yet not bulkier, after just 12 weeks of lifting. Next excuse?

Training Tip

Don't neglect your strength training program when you're away from your usual routine. When I'm traveling and don't have access to weights or machines, I do exercises such as push-ups and pull-ups.

Essential Strengthening Exercises for Runners

As with the stretching routine I laid out in the preceding chapter, the purpose of this section is to show you the minimum of what I think you should do in strength training, not present a one-size-fits-all strength training program. You might have noticed that everything I've said so far about strengthening exercises refers to upper body work. That's what I'm going to focus on here. I'm not saying that runners can't benefit from doing resistance training for their legs, just that I don't think that doing so is as necessary for all runners as the upper body work.

Footnotes

Some top runners have devised innovative strength training routines. In her training before she won the 1992 Los Angeles Marathon, Madina Biktagirova routinely pushed a car to build total body strength. Emil Zatopek, an Olympic gold medalist in the 1950s, used to run while carrying his wife piggyback.

Later on in this chapter, I'll show you a few leg exercises that you might have reason to do, but for now, I'm going to stick to my keep-it-simple mantra. All runners should do some form of strengthening exercises for these areas:

➤ Abdominal muscles
➤ Back

➤ Biceps

➤ Shoulders

➤ Chest

➤ Triceps

These key upper body parts contribute to running more smoothly. When these areas are stronger, you'll be better able to maintain good running form when you get tired.

In some of the exercises that follow, I use small dumbbells. For years, I've used 12-pounders. Again, this is the kind of weight that Arnold Schwarzenegger probably picks his teeth with. That's fine. I'm just working at maintaining a decent level of upper body strength that will help in my running. Those 12-pound dumbbells are what work for me. Find a weight that you can use comfortably throughout the exercises.

Regardless of whatever weight you use, follow these guidelines in your strength training program:

➤ Use a weight that you can comfortably lift 12 times.

➤ After you do all the exercises, relax for a few minutes, and then repeat the set.

➤ Do this workout two or three times a week.

➤ Don't lift weights on consecutive days.

➤ Schedule your strength training sessions for your easier running days or for days when you don't run.

➤ If you have the time, do these workouts after you do your stretching routine.

➤ Do these exercises in the same comfortable clothes that you do your stretching in.

➤ Do the floor exercises on the same firm, comfortable surface that you stretch on.

Keep these guidelines in mind as you review the basic exercises on the following pages.

Training Tip

If you do your strength training at a time other than right after your run, do something to limber up a bit before delving into the exercises. One good way is to work through the exercises you'll be doing with little or no weight for resistance.

Rules of the Road

Wear shoes when you do your strengthening work so that you'll be less likely to slip and hurt yourself.

Crunches

As shown in the following figure, lie on the floor with your back and head flat against the floor to begin the crunches. Bend your knees so that your heels rest on the floor. Cross your arms across your stomach. While keeping your back straight and your butt on the floor, slowly raise your upper body until your shoulders are level with your knees. Try not to curl your upper body toward your knees; instead, imagine that it's being pulled by a string toward the ceiling. Slowly lower your upper body until your back is flat on the floor. Repeat this exercise 25 times.

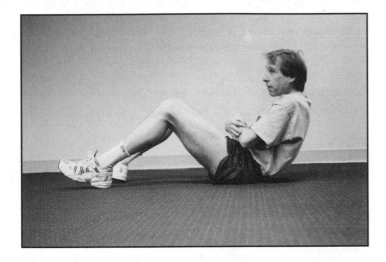

Crunches work your abdominal muscles.

Back Strengthening

To begin the back strengtheningexercise, lie down with your stomach and thighs against the floor, as illustrated in the figure. Prop yourself up on one elbow with your upper arm at a 90-degree angle to the floor, keeping the opposing leg straight and flat. Raise the other arm and the opposing leg to shoulder level at the same time. Hold for a few seconds, then relax and repeat the exercise with the other arm and leg. Do this exercise 10 times with each set of opposing arms and legs.

Back strengthening.

Bicep Curls

To strengthen your biceps, stand straight with a small dumbbell in the palm of one hand. The hand with the weight should rest against your thigh with your palm facing away from you. Using your elbow as a lever, slowly raise the dumbbell to shoulder height, as shown in the figure. Return to the start position just as slowly. Try not to hoist the weight by jerking your shoulder or upper arm. Do 12 repetitions of this exercise for each arm.

Doing curls strengthens your biceps.

Shoulder Press

To begin the shoulder press, stand straight with a small dumbbell in one hand. The arm with the weight should be bent so that the palm of your hand is facing away from you and the weight is roughly at shoulder height, as shown in the following figure. Straighten your arm and slowly push the weight toward the ceiling. Slowly return to the starting position. Repeat the exercise 12 times for each arm.

Shoulder press.

Chest Strengthening

Lie down with your back flat, your knees bent, and your feet on the floor to get in position for the chest strengthening exercise. Keep one arm against your side. In the other, hold a small dumbbell while extending the arm perpendicular to your torso, as shown in the following figure. Slowly raise the weight until it's over your chest, and then slowly lower it to the starting position. Repeat this exercise 12 times for each arm.

Chest strengthening.

Triceps Strengthening

To begin the triceps strengthening exercise, lie on the floor with your back flat, your knees bent and your feet on the ground. Grip a small dumbbell with both hands. Rest your arms on your torso so that the weight is lying near your waist. While keeping your arms straight, slowly pull the weight behind you until it touches the floor behind your head, as shown in the figure. Slowly return to the starting position. Do this exercise 12 times.

Triceps strengthening.

Get the Imbalance Right

Some runners should also do simple leg strengthening exercises. These runners are people who are susceptible to one of three common *muscle imbalances* that can occur between *opposing muscle groups* in the legs: the hamstrings and quadriceps; the calves and shins; and the adductors and abductors. Read on to see whether you have one of these imbalances.

Upper Leg Equilibrium

Ideally, your quadriceps (your thigh muscles) should be about 25 percent stronger than your hamstrings. In other words, if you were to go to a gym, you should be able to lift 25 percent more when doing leg extensions (which work the quadriceps) than when doing leg curls (which work the hamstrings). But running can overdevelop your hamstrings while doing relatively nothing for your quads. An imbalance in the strength ratio between the two muscles might show up as chronic knee pain because the tendons around the knee can become strained by having to work extra hard to compensate for tight, too-strong hamstrings and relatively weak quads. When your quads are stronger, they can absorb more of running's impact shock that is otherwise distributed to the knees.

If you have an imbalance in this area, try this at-home remedy. Fill a gym bag with shoes. While sitting on a chair, dangle the straps of the bag across the top of one foot. Lift the bag by straightening that leg. Do this exercise 12 times for each leg.

Below-the-Knee Balance

As with your hamstrings and quadriceps, your calves may get too strong and tight while your shins get relatively weaker when you run regularly. You might have this imbalance if you have chronic Achilles tendon problems. To strengthen your shin muscles, write the alphabet in the air with your big toe. It sounds strange, but try it. You'll feel right away how effective this exercise can be.

Thigh Therapy

Thigh muscle imbalances happen to the best of us. Long-time runners are more susceptible to this imbalance than are beginners because with a lot of running, the abductor muscles (on the outside of your upper thigh) get stronger while the adductors (on your inner thighs) aren't worked all that much. The problem is that these muscles are supposed to rotate your hips through a full range of motion, so when the adductors become too weak, and the abductors have to do too much work and you get hip pain. If you have this problem, strengthen your adductors by sitting on a chair with a soccer ball between your thighs and squeezing the ball several times.

Training Tip
If you belong to a gym, ask a fitness instructor about exercises on machines that work the same muscles I'm recommending you focus on. For example, using a leg extension machine is a good way to strengthen your quadriceps.

The Least You Need to Know

➤ You'll run more smoothly and with less effort if you regularly do some basic upper body strengthening.

➤ You only need to do strengthening exercises two or three times a week.

➤ The types of strengthening exercises that runners should do aren't the kind that will make you add unwanted bulk.

➤ Runners should concentrate on exercises that strengthen the abdominals, back, arms, and shoulders.

➤ Some runners should do leg strengthening exercises to correct muscle imbalances that can lead to injury.

Chapter 12

The Aches and the Pains

In This Chapter

➤ Why runners get injured

➤ Preventing running injuries

➤ Treating running injuries

➤ The best doctors to see for running injuries

Being injured is the pits. Many times, you can't run at all. Even if you can run with your injury, you usually have to cut back on your usual distance and slow down. Your running just isn't as much fun. Suddenly, your running, which is supposed to help with the stress in your life, adds to it.

Unfortunately, injuries are a part of the sport, and a common one at that. By some estimates, more than half of all runners are injured enough every year to have their training interrupted for more than a week. Now that I've completely depressed you, here's the good news—injuries are common, but they're usually predictable and preventable.

Most running injuries come from trying to do too much too soon at too quick a pace and ignoring the body's signals that it's on overload. So before looking at how to treat common running injuries, I'm going to show you how to avoid them. I hope that after reading the first part of this chapter, you never have reason to read the second.

Are Injuries Inevitable?

One runner I know suffered a broken rib when he tripped during a run. Another I know broke his arm when he didn't see a low chain-link fence during a dark morning run. And while working on this book, my co-author, Scott Douglas, tripped over a dog leash while running and landed on his kneecap so hard that he could barely run for more than a month.

Track Talk
Most running injuries are *overuse injuries*. These injuries occur gradually as a muscle, tendon, ligament, or, more rarely, bone repeatedly has to absorb more shock or work through a greater range of motion than it's prepared to.

These are freak occurrences. They sound like the kinds of injuries that skiers and football players get—random, acute events. Most running injuries, in contrast, are *overuse injuries*—they stem from repeatedly stressing an overworked body part and ignoring the early warning signs that something is wrong.

Why do runners get injured? Remember, when you run, your bones, muscles, tendons, and ligaments deal with forces of at least three times your body weight with each step. In order to continue running, your tissues must be able to withstand these loads, even when they're repeated thousands of times per day. An injury is a failure in your body to handle these repetitive forces.

What causes muscle strains, tendinitis, ligament damage, and stress fractures? Either the forces to which body parts are subjected are too high, or they're repeated too many times. In other words, injuries occur because of too much impact shock with each step, the cumulative effect of too many steps, or a combination of the two.

Most running injuries occur because of the repetitive nature of the running stride. When repeated thousands of time per run, even a slight imperfection in how your feet roll through the gait cycle, for example, can lead to problems nearly anywhere in your legs. That's why you need to take a global view of a running injury—you want to look at not only the area that's bothering you, but what about your running is causing that area to hurt.

Conquering your injury, then, means two things: treating the immediate symptoms, and figuring out what went wrong to cause them. Take care of the symptoms, and you get to start running normally again. Figure out and eliminate the root causes, and you're more likely not to be sidelined by that injury again.

Even if you're not injured, you should always be thinking about how to prevent injuries. Good running habits are so important, because the majority of running injuries can be prevented by eliminating the root causes. To eliminate these root causes, you need to increase the ability of your tissues to tolerate a force repeatedly and/or decrease the cumulative amount of force.

You can increase the ability of your tissues to tolerate repeated forces by doing the following:

1. Regularly stretching the major muscles, tendons, and ligaments that are worked when you run.

2. Correcting muscle imbalances that require a given body part to work harder when you run than it's designed to (see Chapter 12 for how to correct muscle imbalances).

3. Increasing your mileage and intensity gradually so that your body has a chance to adapt to an increased workload.

Be sure to read Chapter 10, "Stretching: the Truth," carefully if you're regularly bothered by soft-tissue (muscle and tendon) injuries.

The second main way to prevent running injuries is to regularly reduce the cumulative amount of shock that you subject your body to. Among the ways to do that are the following:

1. Running on soft surfaces, such as dirt and grass, whenever possible.

2. Running in shoes that have adequate cushioning and that have extra cushioning in the appropriate place if you land hard on a certain part of your foot.

3. Running the appropriate number of miles to meet your goals, not just mindlessly amassing miles. Even the best-constructed body will eventually break down with too many miles.

You'll also reduce the amount of shock to your body if you run at an appropriate weight. Beginning runners who might be overweight should therefore be especially careful about running on soft surfaces in well-cushioned shoes.

Training Tip
A good mental outlook is crucial to conquering an injury. When I have a little injury that's interrupting my training, I tell myself that overcoming it is the most important aspect of my running for the time being. Make getting better your next short-term goal and track your progress toward meeting it as you would any other goal.

Should You Run on It?

Judgment calls are a big part of being a runner. You're always weighing a seemingly endless number of issues in trying to answer some basic questions, such as how far, how fast, and when and where to run. If you're injured, there's an even more basic question to consider: Should you run? Here's where injuries can get the most tricky. If you don't run on your injury, it's not going to bother you. Push this logic to its extreme, and it'll never bother you—never run, and I can guarantee you that you'll never have a running injury.

The standard medical advice for all injuries used to be: Don't run for two weeks. If it bothers you when you start again, take another two weeks off, and keep doing so until you're better. That's not very helpful advice for most running injuries. If all runners stopped running every time they got a little ache or pain, some of them would almost never run!

What you want to know is how to finesse your ache or pain so that you can keep running without doing more damage. After all, a little knot in your calf that loosens up after 10 minutes of easy running is a lot different from an aching hip that makes you limp around the office, and then only gets worse when you try to run on it. How much and whether you should run with your injury depends on how it feels not only when you run, but also the rest of the day.

Rules of the Road
It's OK to run with aches, especially those that lessen as you run. But never run with pain, especially if it worsens as you run.

Track Talk
Anti-inflammatories are drugs that help to reduce swelling. Most running injuries feature inflammation of soft body tissues, so if you can reduce the swelling, then you'll speed recovery and have less pain. Just be sure that you take them to reduce, not mask, pain. The most popular over-the-counter anti-inflammatories are aspirin and ibuprofen.

Although there aren't hard and fast rules for running while injured, here are some general guidelines:

➤ If you don't notice any pain during your run, but have pain after a run or when you get up in the morning, it's OK to run your usual run at your usual pace.

➤ If you notice pain during your run, but it doesn't interfere with your normal running form, it's OK to keep running, but stay close to home so that you can get back quickly if things deteriorate.

➤ If the pain becomes worse the longer you run, limit your running to however long you can run before this deterioration starts.

➤ If the pain causes you to alter your usual running form, don't run with this injury until you can run normally at a relaxed pace. Running differently because of an injury will make other body parts more susceptible to injury, because they're being asked to work harder than usual to compensate for the injured part that you're favoring.

➤ If your pain interferes with your normal, day-to-day nonrunning activities, the only running you should even think about doing is to the nearest sports medicine doctor's office.

If you're injured and can run, or even if you just feel the beginnings of an injury, try to run primarily on flat surfaces. Running downhill increases the pounding on your legs, and running uphill forces your tendons and muscles to work extra hard. When you're already flirting with disaster, you don't need either. In all of these cases, consider taking *anti-inflammatories* and applying ice to the painful area a few times a day.

Running Hot and Cold

Ice should always be your first line of defense against injury. If I notice the slightest little ache, I like to ice it after my run and a couple of other times during the day, too, if possible. A few minutes of preventative care can work wonders in keeping a little nagging pain from developing into a disruptive injury.

Why ice instead of heat? The reason is that most running injuries are a result of soft body tissues (muscles, tendons, ligaments) that have become inflamed. Blood vessels get damaged and swell; the greater the swelling, the worse the injury, and the longer recovery is going to take. Icing the inflamed area causes the blood vessels to constrict. This reduces the swelling because less blood flows to the injured area and the damaged tissue relaxes.

This not only reduces the pain you feel, but also speeds healing, because as the tissue's metabolism is slowed, there's less tissue breakdown. Heating an inflamed area worsens, rather than improves things. Heat has the opposite effect of ice, so the blood vessels of the injured area become that much more swollen.

Heat is helpful when your inflammation has reduced, however. This reduction usually won't occur for at least 72 hours. At this point, the increased blood flow that heating stimulates will speed delivery of nutrients to the damaged tissue, thereby speeding healing. Heat is also good if you have overall stiffness in an area. The general rule is to use ice on small, acute body aches because they are signs of damage to a specific body part and to use heat for more widespread stiffness.

Always ice an injury for at least 5, but no more than 20 minutes. The area should become red and numb, not white and numb. After running is the best time to ice, because the tissues will be the most swollen, but you'll speed recovery if you can find a few other times during the day to ice. Rub the ice in circular motions on the injured body part.

The best method of icing I've found is to fill a few paper cups with water and keep them in your freezer. When you need to ice an injury, just tear down the top

Rules of the Road
Don't heat an area for more than 20 minutes at a time. Otherwise, you're risking a burn.

Training Tip
If you have a large area to ice, consider creating an ice wrap. A bag of small, frozen vegetables, such as peas and corn, is good for this. Another solution to keep a mixture of three parts water to one part alcohol in a bag in the freezer. Because the alcohol won't freeze, the bag will have some give to it.

of the cup until the ice is exposed and hold the cup from the bottom while icing. This method keeps your hands warm while you ice, so you're more likely to stick with it for the proper amount of time. When you're done icing your injury, just put the cup back in the freezer until you need it again. These cups can last for months and will ensure that you always have one handy.

The Agony of Da Feet

Most people would say that runners have nice bodies, or at least they would until they got a look at runners' feet. Your feet can take a lot of abuse, and all that pounding and sliding around and sweating can cause quite a stink if left unattended. More important than looks, some runner's feet develop problems that can sideline them from more than the "World's Prettiest Toes" contest.

Tending to Toes

Most toe problems you're going to get as a runner are cosmetic rather than serious. The most frequent visitors will be black toenails, which are so linked with the sport that the condition is also known as runner's toe. Runner's toe happens when the nail is either pressed down too much on the bed that underlies it or the nail separates from the bed. In either case, blood pools between the nail and the bed. Eventually, the nail turns black.

When this condition is caused by the nail being pressed into the bed, it's almost never painful. The nail gets very hard, and it looks like hell, but it won't bother you. After a few months, the nail will grow out or fall off. In the meantime, you've got yourself a nice little memento from your miles that will instantly identify you as a runner to any knowledgeable person who happens to see your feet.

Sometimes, the nail loosens rather than hardens, and this is usually uncomfortable. New runners whose toenails aren't used to much wear and tear will get these more than long-time runners. If your black toenail is wobbly, sterilize a needle, and then use it to drain the blood from under the nail, as you would drain a blister.

Runner's toe is usually caused by ill-fitting shoes. If your shoes aren't long enough, your longest toe (which in some people is the second toe) will slam against the front of the shoe. You might also irritate your nails by running on a course that has a lot more downhills than you're used to, because your toes are going to rise up a bit more than usual on the downhills to help you brake. Wet shoes, either from sweat or rain, are also a leading cause of runner's toe.

Poorly fitting shoes may also cause blisters, "hot spots," and other irritations on the tops of your toes. When a pair of shoes causes blisters during your first few runs, then you've probably bought shoes that are too small. Cover these irritated spots with one of the many second-skin products on the market, and you'll usually be fine.

Healing Your Heels

The most common running injury to the heel area is called plantar fasciitis. This condition is an inflammation of the plantar fascia, a fibrous band of tissue that runs from the heel to the toes. You'll feel pain along the inside bottom of your foot anywhere from the heel through the arch. Many times, the pain is worst when you step out of bed in the morning or when you've been sitting for a long time, and then it improves during the day as the plantar fascia has a chance to loosen up.

The plantar fascia most often becomes inflamed because it has to work through more of a range of motion than it's designed to. When your heel strikes the ground, the pressure on the heel pulls on the plantar fascia. If your calf muscles are too tight, or if you overpronate but don't wear shoes with enough motion control, then you're most likely to develop plantar fasciitis. Also, high-arched, rigid feet can predispose you to this injury because when your heel lands, your foot doesn't move enough, so the plantar fascia has to absorb more shock.

Footnotes

There's great variation even among top runners in injury rate. In the last 30 years, I've had only one injury that has plagued me for more than a month (a case of plantar fasciitis soon after I turned 40). Contrast that with Mary Slaney, who used to hold every American record from 800 meters to 10K. Despite being light and having textbook running form, she's very fragile and claims not to be able to remember how many times she's had surgery!

The best treatment for plantar fasciitis is icing. Ice the bottom of your foot from heel to ball. One good trick is to ice your foot with a frozen cola bottle (if you can still find the glass ones). The cold of the bottle does the work of the ice, and rolling your foot over the contours of the bottle gives the plantar fascia a nice little massage. (It's pretty hard to stretch it otherwise.)

Most people with plantar fasciitis can run on the injury. Cut back if the pain gets worse, not better, as you run. Preventative steps include increasing the flexibility of your calves and Achilles tendons, and making sure that your shoes have the proper combination of motion control and cushioning.

Stressed Out

Stress fractures are tiny, incomplete breaks or cracks in a bone. They can occur many places in the body, but runners most often get them in the feet. They're caused by too much repetitive stress to bones that are overworked. That's why stress fractures occur gradually—over time, the bones are asked to do just a little bit more than they're ready for, and the shock is great enough to cause a slight crack.

Stress fractures are different from a standard broken bone because with a stress fracture, there's not a sudden, obvious incident when the bone breaks. Rather, the pain begins gradually, usually as a slight twinge, and only intensifies as you continue to run on it. Trust me, though—if you get a full-blown stress fracture, there will be no mistaking that you're hurt. With every step, sharp pain will shoot from your foot up your leg, and it will get worse the longer you run on it.

Stress fractures are almost always caused by some of the errors that I outlined earlier in this chapter—increasing mileage and intensity too quickly, wearing shoes without enough cushioning, and doing too much of your running on hard surfaces. Runners who don't include enough calcium in their diets are also susceptible.

Training Tip

When you're coming back from an injury, err on the side of caution. The last thing you want to do is come back too quickly and re-trigger your injury. If you had to take some time off, allow twice as much time as you were off to build back to your regular mileage.

Unfortunately, when you have a stress fracture, you need to stop running. Otherwise, you're just asking for it. The bone will continue to rupture, and you could develop a complete break, which will add considerably to your downtime. So if you feel the beginnings of a stress fracture, take a few days off and ice the area (which will probably be a little tender and swollen, and maybe even a bit warm to the touch at first). If you definitely have a stress fracture, you're best off not running for at least two weeks, as well as avoiding other weight-bearing activity during this time. If it's still bad when you restart, stop again, and see a doctor.

Leggings

Continuing our tour up the trail of woe, let's look at running injuries that you feel above the feet. Bear in mind that although these injuries occur above the foot, they are usually caused by something that goes wrong at footstrike.

Achilles' Last Stand

The Achilles' heel for some runners is the Achilles tendon. That's because the Achilles tendon—a cord-like structure that connects the heel to the calf muscles—has a fairly limited range of motion. It can get overworked pretty easily. To make matters worse, blood flow to the area is poor, so it takes a while to get loosened up.

If you have Achilles tendinitis, you'll know it because nothing else causes sharp pain in that area. The pain, which can also be a burning sensation, will be anywhere from an inch above your heel to the bottom of your calf. In bad cases, you'll be able to see how inflamed the tendon is, because it will be visibly swollen compared to your healthy Achilles tendon.

Achilles tendinitis is often caused by many of the same things that lead to plantar fasciitis, including tight calf muscles and overpronation. Sometimes it can be caused when the back of your shoe sits too high against your heel. (This is why you'll see many running shoes with notches at the top of the heel counter.)

In addition to the standards of icing, anti-inflammatories, and cutting back on your running if your normal form is altered, here's another trick for beating Achilles tendinitis: Wear heel lifts in your street and running shoes until the problem goes away. The lifts will take some of the pressure off your inflamed tendon by elevating it. A simple, at-home method is to cut a half-circle that fits your heel from corrugated cardboard. Be sure to put a new one in at least once a day as the cardboard gets compressed. In the long term, be extra careful about stretching, and get out of the habit of wearing high-heeled shoes, which can shorten and tighten your calves and Achilles tendons.

Stopping Shin Splints

Shin splints—or what the running doctors call tibial stress syndrome—are one of the most common injuries for new runners. That's because they're usually caused by muscle and tendon weakness in the front or inside of the lower leg. With more running, these areas become strong enough to handle the increased stress they're being subjected to. Weak arches can also lead to shin splints by making the shin muscles work extra hard to raise your arches when you run. Shin splints can lead to stress fractures, so you want to beat them before they beat you.

Shin splints are tiny tears of the front lower leg muscles away from the shin bone (or tibia). At first, you might notice a pulling or vague aching sensation in the area after you run. The pain can become sharp, usually after you've run for a certain amount of time. The area around the shin may become inflamed, or lumps may form where the muscle tries to reattach itself.

I don't mean to sound like a broken record here, but the best immediate treatment for shin splints is the standard: ice, anti-inflammatories, and cutting back on your mileage. And another thing I keep harping on: Run on soft surfaces whenever possible. Shin splints are one of those injuries that people sensitive to running's pounding get; that's why beginners, who haven't built up as much resistance to pounding, get them much more frequently than long-timers. So reduce that pounding by running on more forgiving ground.

The Knee Bone's Connected to the...

The fear that most people have of runners' knees—crippling arthritis—is largely unfounded. That doesn't mean that runners don't get knee injuries, though. In fact, in one survey of runners, injuries to the knee were more common than injuries to any other body part.

Let's face it: The knee is one of the most poorly "designed" parts of our body. This tiny little shifting piece of bone acts as the brace between our feet crashing into the ground and almost the entire rest of our body. Add to that the stress of running on asphalt, overpronation, and, for some, being overweight, and it's a wonder that there aren't more knee injuries!

Footnotes

Whenever you start to despair that your running injury is erasing all of your hard-won fitness, remember this: In 1984, Joan Benoit Samuelson won the Olympic Marathon trials just 17 days after having arthroscopic surgery on her knee. This is an extreme case, but many runners try to view an injury as an enforced rest period that will increase their motivation to do well when they've recuperated.

The two most common knee injuries for runners are iliotibial band syndrome and, appropriately enough, runner's knee (what the professionals call chondromalacia patella). As explained in Chapter 10, the iliotibial band is a thick cord that runs from the pelvis to the outside of the thigh and connects just below the knee. It helps to stabilize your thigh muscles and knee when you run. Usually, you'll feel pain on the outside of your knee, but you might also feel it along the outside of your hip. The pain can be sporadic from day to day, but it usually comes on after you've run a set distance.

Bowlegged runners are susceptible to this injury. They should concentrate on regularly stretching the iliotibial band to make sure that it can work through a wide enough range of motion when running. And anyone can get it if they regularly run on uneven surfaces, especially the same side of an overly slanted road.

In the short term, you're best to limit your mileage to just below the level at which you usually start to feel pain. In the long term, be smart—work on increasing the band's flexibility, and run on level surfaces. If you have no option but to run on slanted roads, regularly switch directions so that one leg isn't always made to run as if it were longer.

In runner's knee, repeated stress on the knee causes inflammation and softening of the cartilage under the kneecap. This prevents the kneecap from tracking normally over the end of the thigh bone. You'll usually feel pain around or behind the kneecap; it might get worse when you climb stairs.

Overpronators are especially susceptible to runner's knee because the knee has to compensate for the extra inward rotation of the lower leg. Among relatively new runners, weak thigh muscles are often a leading cause of this injury. Your thigh muscles help to align your knee and keep it straight. If they're not as strong as they should be, they may not be able to help the knee guide itself along its proper course.

In addition to icing the entire area around your knee, you can get some relief from runner's knee by avoiding steep downhills, uneven surfaces, and other factors that are going to require your knee to do extra work to stabilize itself. (You also might want to avoid the tight turns of indoor tracks.) If you're repeatedly bothered by pain around your kneecap, get running shoes with better motion control.

Don't Get Hamstrung

Long-time runners suffer from injuries in the hamstring, hip, and buttock area more than beginners. Many of us have seen sprinters pull up suddenly with a hamstring tear. That doesn't happen very often to distance runners. Our hamstring problems are low-grade, chronic microtears that accumulate over time and usually because of neglect. Most of these injuries are the result of poor flexibility in these areas, and veteran runners who don't have good stretching habits are notoriously tight from knee to butt.

But beware of hamstring problems if your job involves long periods of sitting. Sitting for long periods can shorten your hamstrings and the surrounding muscles and tendons. Try not to sit for more than an hour at a time. In your runs, ease into your normal pace to give the large muscles along the back of your legs a chance to warm up.

Which Doctors to Run To

When should you see a doctor for a running injury? Most injuries, especially the soft-tissue overuse injuries, don't need medical attention, especially if you treat them right from the start. When an injury drags on, or when you keep running on it and you get injured elsewhere, you start entering the gray area of when to get help. Certainly, any runner whose injury interferes with normal, daily activity for more than a week without improvement should seek medical help.

If your injury is a problem only when you run, then when and how soon to see a doctor is up to you. If your self-care routine doesn't seem to be working, then you should probably see a doctor who might be able to diagnose and treat the underlying cause. Runners can be pretty stubborn in their self-reliance, but sometimes you just have to bite the medical bullet and admit that your problem isn't getting better on its own. Deciding to go to the doctor often comes down to how willing you are to put up with the lack of enjoyment that your running injury is causing you.

Rules of the Road

If you have a slight muscle tear, don't vigorously stretch the area; doing so might increase the inflammation. It's better to exercise it gently to increase the flow of blood and healing nutrients to the area.

You should also see a doctor if you repeatedly get injured in the same small part of your body. This type of injury means that you have an underlying weakness or structural deformity. A good sports medicine doctor will be able to get to the root of the problem so that the area won't plague you throughout your running career.

Notice that I said a sports medicine doctor. Fortunately, the last 20 years of the fitness boom have produced a growth in the number of sports medicine doctors, who specialize in treating athletes. These doctors have the training, experience, and mindset to look at your injury as you do—an interruption of your body's normal way of operating that needs to be treated at its root, not just for its symptoms.

Footnotes

How about seeing these guys for a sympathetic ear about your running injuries? Tony Sandavol, who won the 1980 Olympic Marathon trials, and Bob Kempainen, who won the 1996 Olympic Marathon trials, are both medical doctors.

How do you find a good sports medicine doctor? As always, word of mouth from other runners is the best way. Some doctors belong to professional organizations for sports medicine doctors, but not all. Also, the American Running and Fitness Association maintains a listing of more than 5,000 of these professionals throughout the country. To find one in your area, call (800) 776-ARFA.

In general, avoid doctors who do the following:

➤ Propose that you stop running as the final solution

➤ Treat only your symptoms, rather than looking for the cause of your problem

➤ Say they don't have much experience working with athletes

➤ Don't look at surgery as a last resort

Of course, most insurance plans are going to require a referral to see a specialist, so you might have to have an initial meeting with someone who acts this way. But once you get to a specialist, make sure that he or she thinks differently.

What types of specialists should runners see? That depends on your injury. Foot and lower leg injuries can be treated by orthopedists or osteopaths (I'll say more about them in a minute), but they're most often treated by podiatrists. Podiatrists have the initials D.P.M. (doctor of podiatric medicine) following their name. Podiatrists complete four years of training at a college of podiatric medicine and a residency. They are licensed to perform surgery and prescribe medicine.

Podiatrists focus not only on feet, but also on problems elsewhere that are caused by feet. This focus makes them among the runner's best medical friends, because so many running injuries are caused by faulty feet. A podiatrist can determine whether factors such as overpronation or weak arches are contributing to problems in your biomechanics and setting you up for injury. These types of structural problems in the feet are often treated with *orthotics*. Podiatrists are the best professionals to see to determine if you need orthotics, and they're trained to cast the devices for you.

Knee injuries are most often treated by orthopedists, although some knee problems are caused by problems in your feet and can therefore be addressed by podiatrists. Orthopedists are medical doctors (M.D.s) who treat injuries to bones, muscles, tendons, and ligaments. Orthopedists have a reputation for performing surgery, and although a good sports medicine orthopedist will always favor more conservative treatment first, many runners are leery of seeing orthopedists for this reason.

> **Track Talk**
> *Orthotics* are devices worn in shoes to combat an underlying structural problem in the feet. They're usually prescribed by a podiatrist. Hard orthotics help to limit your foot's motion, so they are made for overpronators. Soft orthotics are made for people with rigid feet to help absorb and distribute some of the pounding of running.

Running injuries above the knee are also often treated by orthopedists. Another good type of doctor to see for these ailments is an osteopath. Like M.D.s, osteopaths (D.O.s) are licensed to practice all branches of medicine, prescribe medication, and perform surgery. In general, they're trained to view the body more systematically, so they're likely to look at a runner's injury from the standpoint of unearthing the root cause rather than just treating the symptoms.

Each of these three specialties has a professional sports medicine organization:

➤ The American Academy of Podiatric Sports Medicine (301) 424-7440

➤ The American Orthopedic Society for Sports Medicine (708) 292-4900

➤ The American Osteopathic Academy of Sports Medicine (608) 831-4400

I'm not saying that these are the only types of medical professionals that runners can benefit from seeing. Chiropractors (D.C.s), physiatrists (M.D.s trained similarly to osteopaths), physical therapists (P.T.s), and others can also be helpful. But podiatrists, orthopedists, and osteopaths are usually going to be the first ones to see for most common running injuries.

The Least You Need to Know

➤ Most running injuries are caused by overuse and can be prevented.

➤ Increasing mileage gradually, running on soft surfaces, and having good stretching and strengthening habits are some of the best ways to prevent injuries.

➤ Most running injuries will go away with a combination of rest and conservative treatment.

➤ Apply ice, not heat, to new running injuries.

➤ A trip to the doctor isn't necessary for most running injuries.

➤ If you have to see a doctor, which one is best depends on what type of injury you have. Seek out a sports medicine doctor for the best diagnosis and treatment.

Eating on the Run: Deciding on Your Diet

Food is fuel. Even if your main motivation for starting a running program is to lose weight, you're not going to make it very far down the road if your muscles don't have the fuel they need. That fuel comes almost entirely from one source—what you eat.

Unfortunately, that pretty simple concept is misunderstood by scores of runners. Remember what I said in Chapter 10 about how carried away some runners get arguing about stretching? Well that's nothing compared to what you'll hear said about the runner's diet. About the only thing I've ever heard debated as fiercely as what runners should eat was involvement in the Vietnam War when I was in college in the '60s. My goal in this chapter is to cut through all the chatter and state a few dietary facts. By the end of this chapter, you'll know the basics of a good diet for runners and what *isn't* necessary nutritionally.

Do Running Nuts Live on Berries?

As I've said, one of the questions that I'm asked most frequently has to do with whether my knees bother me because of all those miles. Probably the second most popular question I hear is, "You eat *that*?" This question comes about when I'm doing something as innocent as having a cup of coffee. It also happens if I'm enjoying a doughnut, putting cream cheese on a bagel, or having a glass of wine with dinner.

Somewhere along the way, most people got the notion that being a runner means living off of the twigs and nuts that you gather out of your backyard. When running first achieved mass popularity in the '70s, the sport was seen as part of a new movement for Americans who had decided that it was time to take charge of their health. So in the public mind running became associated with health food stores, megavitamin doses, and drinking nothing but carrot juice and purified water.

I think that's too bad. Not because running can't be an incredibly big step toward taking control of your health. No, the problem is that people who are new to running have been led to believe that starting an exercise program also means a simultaneous radical change in your diet. That's not true, and it saddens me that some people might view running as off-putting because of this image.

That doesn't mean that being a runner means eating whatever you want. Yes, I'm as well-known in some circles for my legendary consumption of junk food as I am for my marathon victories. And as I've hinted, I still like to indulge myself occasionally. Eating is one of the major pleasures of life, and who doesn't like to live a little now and then?

Footnotes

My "junk food habit" has gotten a lot of attention over the years, but it's been overplayed. Yes, I have a sweet tooth, and even the legend about me putting mayonnaise on pizza crust is true. But I couldn't have run more than 100 miles a week year after year and have only one serious injury in the last 25 years if there wasn't a good diet underlying those occasional indulgences.

But as you become fitter through your running, you're probably going to be motivated to make changes in other parts of your life that will improve your health, such as getting more sleep and eating better. Running can help you to acquire an appreciation for simpler, heartier foods, which usually fuel you better and don't bother you as much when you run. The upshot is this: Most runners find that they feel better if they make a few simple, healthful changes in their diets. But that doesn't have to entail shopping only at the local organic produce shop. As most long-time runners will tell you, one of the great things about running is that all those miles often mean eating more and not gaining weight.

The Real Runner's Diet

If runners' diets seem strange to most folks, that's because most people don't eat as most nutritionists advise. That's another way of saying that the best diet for runners is the one that everyone should eat. This diet should be low in fat and include a moderate amount of lean, high-quality protein; the majority of calories should come from carbohydrates, especially in the form of fresh fruits and vegetables and whole grains.

More than sedentary people, runners gravitate toward this type of diet because it makes them feel better. As you become fitter, you become more in touch with your body and with how it feels when you put certain things in it. I mean this both in the short term—those slices of bacon just don't seem to taste as good right after a morning run—and long term, as you learn how some foods fuel your running better than others.

Although your diet is important to your overall health, it's not the key to your running; your training is. No amount of dietary manipulation is going to make up for miles logged. A good diet is important because it will allow you to get the most out of your running, not because it's going to make you a better runner.

That statement may seem as though I'm splitting hairs, but I'm not. I've heard a lot of runners before races talk about how they've been eating such and such and not eating such and such, so they know that they'll do well in the race. Then I hear how much they've been running (usually not much), and it's obvious that they think they can eat their way to peak performance. That's a classic American belief—if we just take the right pill, we can avoid having to do the real work—but a unfounded one. A bad diet will probably get in the way of your running, but the most that a good diet will do for you is allow you to reap the results of the training that you do. That said, let's look at the three main sources of calories in everyone's diet: carbohydrates, protein, and fat.

Rules of the Road
Runners should have healthful diets for the simple reason that everyone should. Running doesn't mean that the nutritional rules don't apply to you. There's a history of high cholesterol in my family. About 10 years ago, I was shocked to discover that my cholesterol level was in the 230s, even after so many years of so many miles. Once I made some simple changes to lower my fat intake, my cholesterol level went down.

Carbs: a Runner's Best Friend

Carbohydrates, or just carbs to most runners, are your body's main source of energy for aerobic exercise. One gram of carbohydrate contains four calories. Your body converts the carbohydrates you eat into glucose, a simple sugar. Glucose is then either used immediately by your body for energy or converted to glycogen, which, as Chapter 2 explained, is the fuel stored in the muscles that power your running. When runners "bonk" or "hit The Wall" and have to slow dramatically, they've run out of carbohydrates. (Chapter 22, "In It For the Long Run: The Marathon" discusses this situation.)

Track Talk
Carbohydrates are sugars that fuel your muscles during exercise. You eat them in both complex form (such as pasta) and simple form (such as honey). You should get 60 to 65 percent of your calories from carbohydrates.

Carbohydrates are classified as either complex or simple. This classification has to do not with how philosophical they are, but with how they're constructed chemically. Complex carbohydrates are starches, such as grains, and simple carbohydrates are sugars, such as the fructose found in fruits. Common food sources of carbohydrates include fruits, vegetables, pasta, rice, bread products, cereals, and jellies.

You should aim for 60 to 65 percent of your calories to come from carbohydrates. This amount will keep your muscles well-fueled so that you'll be able to meet your training goals. A high-carb diet chosen from the right sources also means that you're more likely to be getting all of the nutrients that you need because fruits, vegetables, and grains are packed with vitamins and minerals.

Most of the carbohydrates that you eat should be either fruits and vegetables or complex carbs such as pasta. Aim for this level of carbohydrate intake each day:

➤ 10 to 12 servings of grains (one serving equals a slice of bread, half a cup of cooked pasta, half a bagel, or one ounce of cereal)

➤ 5 to 7 servings of fruit (one serving equals a medium-sized piece of fruit, half a grapefruit, or four ounces of juice)

➤ 4 to 5 servings of vegetables (one serving equals one cup raw vegetables or half a cup cooked)

If these amounts seem like a lot, keep in mind how small one serving is. If you pour yourself a decent-sized bowl of cereal, that's probably three or four servings right there. Complete your breakfast with half a banana on your cereal, a slice of toast, and a small glass of juice, and you're already past 5 servings for the day. And that's not counting the carbs in the milk that you put on your cereal.

But aren't starches going to make you fat? No. Starches are complex carbohydrates. They contain four calories per gram, just like the carbohydrates found in fruit and vegetables. If you gain weight from eating a lot of starches, that's from eating more calories than you burn, not because of anything inherently fattening about starches. The reason that people think that starches are fattening is that they're often eaten with high-fat foods that contain a lot of extra calories. You butter your bread, fry your potatoes, or have pizza with sausage and extra cheese.

This kind of misunderstanding shows that it's important to make sure that what you think is a high-carb food really is. When you have a thick crust pizza loaded with veggies, that's high-carb. But when you have the thin crust meat lover's special, more than half of the calories are coming from fat. Other supposed high-carb foods that are usually high in fat include muffins, granola, and macaroni and cheese.

Where's the Beef?

Protein is in every part of your body, from muscles to hair. Protein from your diet helps to build and repair muscles and regulate hormones. If you don't get enough protein, you'll recover from injuries and infections more slowly. One gram of protein contains four calories.

About 15 percent of your calories should come from protein. That's less than most people eat. The recommended amount of protein means two to three servings each day, with a serving size being as small as two ounces of chicken or two teaspoons of peanut butter. Chow down on a half-pounder at your favorite burger place and right there you've exceeded your protein needs for the day. A good guideline to follow is that your servings of protein should be no bigger than a deck of cards.

So for most people, getting 15 percent of their calories from protein is going to mean eating less protein than they're used to. The exceptions are people who restrict their protein intake because they think that it's good nutrition to exist on nothing but bagels, salads, and rice cakes. That's taking things too far the other way.

What's wrong with eating too much protein? It means that you're probably falling short in your carb intake. This shortfall could hurt your running because protein supplies a very small percentage of the energy for your running. Also, unless you choose carefully, the protein that you eat might come in a high-fat package, such as a marbled T-bone steak. Eating extra protein doesn't build bigger muscles any more than eating pig's feet helps you to grow extra toes. Extra protein that you eat mainly gives you very expensive urine.

The Skinny on Fat

Many of us are all too familiar with fat, but fat isn't all bad. With nine calories in a gram, or more than twice the amount of a gram of carbohydrate or protein, it's a concentrated energy source. It's what your body burns at low levels of activity, such as when you're sitting at a desk or walking easily. Fat supplies and transports some vitamins, helps to maintain nerve fibers and cell membranes, insulates you from the cold, and cushions internal organs.

Training Tip
Many runners exclude dairy products from their diets. This is a mistake because low-fat and nonfat dairy products are excellent sources of protein and they provide calcium, which is essential to keeping your bones strong enough to withstand running's pounding. Aim for two to three servings of dairy products a day.

Rules of the Road
Don't go overboard on eating low-fat foods. You need some fat in your diet, not only for essential body functions such as digestion and providing cushioning for organs, but also because fat adds taste and texture to your meals. Also, many manufactured nonfat foods, such as pastries, have as many or more calories per serving than the foods they're meant to replace.

In a good diet, 20 to 25 percent of your calories come from fat. This amount is less than most Americans eat—the average is 37 percent of calories from fat. Eating too much fat means that you're not getting the carbs you need to restock your muscles from run to run. It's also bad for your health because a high fat intake has been linked to heart disease and some cancers. And extra fat from your diet is easily stored as extra fat on you.

If you emphasize getting 60 to 65 percent of your calories from carbohydrates, with plenty of fruits and vegetables in the mix, it will be easier to get your fat intake into the 20 to 25 percent range. Choosing lean cuts of protein, such as white chicken meat instead of a greasy cheese steak sub, also helps.

Putting It All Together

Worrying about this percentage of carbohydrates and that percentage of fats sounds like a lot of work. How can you reasonably eat this way without taking a calculator with you on every trip to the kitchen? And what about when you eat out? Relax. The key to a good runner's diet isn't math, but making the right food choices. After all, a meal of butter, beef jerky, and cola can supply you with the right amounts of carbohydrate, protein, and fat, but it's a disaster nutritionally.

Concentrate on getting the number of servings for each food type that I've emphasized. The percentages will take care of themselves if you focus on a variety of wholesome carbohydrates, fruits and vegetables, low-fat dairy products, lean cuts of meat, and legumes. Here's a tip: carbohydrates, such as whole grains, vegetables, and beans, should cover most of the space on your dinner plate. Protein should be the accompaniment, not the centerpiece that many people make it. This guideline is true both at home and when you eat out.

Training Tip
Don't forget the most important thing to consume on a regular basis—water. Drink at least 10 eight-ounce glasses of water a day, plus however much you lose sweating on your runs.

Following these guidelines requires a big change in eating habits for many people. Two good books on eating for athletes are the *Sports Nutrition Guidebook* by Nancy Clark, Human Kinetics, 1996, and *Power Foods* by Liz Applegate, Rodale Press, 1994. It can also help to consult a registered dietitian. Registered dietitians have the initials R.D. after their names. Contact the local branch of the American Dietetic Association to find one in your area.

Sports Bars and Other Goop

Sports bars or energy bars didn't exist in their current incarnation until 1986. Now one company alone, Powerfood, makers of the market-leading PowerBar, has yearly sales of more than $30 million (see the following figure). Should you add to its new-found wealth?

Invented just more than a decade ago, energy bars and gels now have yearly sales of more than $100 million.

You've probably seen these things. They weigh a few ounces, come in a shiny wrapper, and for the most part, don't taste all that great. So why are so many sold? Several reasons, many having to do with great marketing. The main useful reason is that they provide a couple of hundred of easily digestible calories that your body can use almost immediately for energy.

An increasing number of runners find a use for these products in their busy lives. Runners usually eat these bars within 90 minutes of a run when they're dragging and want something to eat before their run that won't bother them during the run. These bars certainly fit that bill. Runners also eat them soon after a hard or long workout, when they want to get something in their system to speed recovery but can't yet stomach "real" food. Some runners also eat hunks of them on long runs, although the new energy gels are supplanting this use. And for people on the go, they're easy to carry and eat at any time.

No runner *needs* an energy bar, however. After all, Frank Shorter had already won his second Olympic Marathon medal 10 years before the first energy bar was sold. As an example, a Malt-Nut PowerBar contains 225 calories, with 83 percent of them from carbohydrate, 10 percent of calories from protein, and 7 percent from fat. It sells for about $1.30. Eaten together, a bagel and a banana contain 275 calories, with 84 percent of them from carbs and 8 percent each from protein and fat. They taste better than energy bars to most people, are just as convenient, and cost about half as much.

> ### Rules of the Road
> Energy bars are usually fortified with vitamins and minerals, but this isn't a reason to eat them. You shouldn't use energy bars or any other fortified product to try to make up for a poor diet. Get your vitamins and minerals from naturally occurring sources. If you choose to eat energy bars, do so for the real reasons they're made.

The new kid on this block are energy gels. These pudding-like gooey glops are increasingly favored by marathoners, both as something to take for a little extra energy during long training runs and as a performance booster on the run during the race. Costing about $1 each, gels come in plastic containers about the size of a takeout ketchup packet, so they're easy to carry. They're also a lot easier to take on the run than energy bars.

Most gels contain about 100 calories of simple carbohydrates, about the amount that you'll burn in a mile of running. Research has shown that when you're exercising and consume simple carbohydrates such as these, the carbs are absorbed directly into your bloodstream for instant energy. (That's why sport drinks, which I'll say more about in Chapter 16, work well, too.) You need to drink several ounces of water soon after consuming a gel to help its absorption. If you're not carrying fluids with you, time it so that you finish downing your gel soon before you'll have access to liquids, such as a water fountain or aid station in a race.

Footnotes

Sport bars and gels are a big improvement over what runners use to consume in long races. In the early part of this century, it was common to give runners whiskey and brandy late in a marathon!

Who needs energy gels? Technically, nobody—as I said, people did long training runs and marathons before these products were invented. Nonetheless, I've certainly come to appreciate the little mid-run boost I get from a gel during a run. However, I use gels only when I'm going to be running for more than 90 minutes. If you don't run this kind of distance, then save your money.

If you are going to be working up to running for that long, then gels can help you. Plan to eat one when you're about two-thirds of the way through your run, such as 10 miles into a 15-miler. Some runners consume two or more on really long runs. The following table lists the choices you have in both energy gels and sports bars.

Sports Bars and Gels

Bars

Bar	Calories	Carbohydrates
Real Berry Clif Bar	250	52 grams
Peanut Butter Met-RX Bar	340	50 grams
Oatmeal Raisin PowerBar	230	45 grams
Chocolate Praline PR Bar	230	24 grams
Apple Cinnamon VO2 Max Bar	240	47 grams

Gels

Bar	Calories	Carbohydrates
Vanilla Bean Gu	100	25 grams
Chocolate Hammer Gel	100	20 grams
Lemon Lime Pocket Rocket	100	25 grams
Vanilla PowerGel	110	28 grams
Lemon Lime Squeezy	80	20 grams
Ultra Gel	133	24 grams

Popping Pills: Vitamins and Other Supplements

Bee pollen, ginseng, beta carotene, chromium, brewer's yeast—the list of wonder substances that are supposedly going to dramatically improve your health and performance is endless. We Americans are always looking for that magic pill that's going to help us lose weight, feel great, have more energy, and, what the hey, why not have it prevent baldness and improve our sex lives at the same time. But the truth is that you can't eat your way to being fit any more than you can eat your way to a college degree or a successful career. These acheivements all take a lot of steady, hard, and sometimes not terribly exciting work. Yet the nutritional supplement industry, to the tune of more than $4 billion a year, has somehow convinced people that health and fitness can be achieved differently.

Vitamins and other supplements are often marketed as energy boosters or some such vague claim. Problem is, vitamins and minerals don't provide energy. Food does. More specifically, the calories in food do. Only foods and drinks that contain calories provide energy.

What do vitamins and minerals do, then? Vitamins are like your body's spark plugs—they are catalysts to reactions within your body. Minerals are elements that form and regulate the body. If your car wasn't firing properly, you might get the spark plugs fixed. But once you got your spark plugs up to normal operating level, you wouldn't throw four more under the hood and expect your car to run better. You would just be wasting your money with your misunderstanding of what keeps your car moving down the road day after day.

Same thing goes for taking vitamins beyond the base level needed for good health. No studies have found increased performance in runners who take megadoses compared to runners who have a normal intake. In fact, no studies have shown increased performance caused by any of these kinds of supplements, be they vitamins, minerals, or substances not even recognized as necessary for normal human functioning, such as bee pollen. The right nutrition for good performance is pretty much the same as it is for good health, regardless of your level of activity.

Most nutritionists would say that it's OK to take a daily multivitamin as a sort of health insurance, but even that shouldn't be necessary if you regularly eat a wide variety of healthful foods. Vitamins and minerals from food are always better than the same substances from pills. When you get vitamins and minerals from food, you're more likely to regularly be eating properly. For example, getting enough vitamin C from your diet means that you're eating a decent amount of fresh fruits and vegetables. Having to meet your vitamin C needs with a pill means that you're going to be hurting in other areas nutritionally, such as fiber and other disease-protective substances best found in food.

Knowing all this information, I still find myself nearly getting hoodwinked once in a while by some smooth talker who promises the key to feeling great. The idea that taking pill X will solve all of your problems is just so appealing. When you hear claims like this, try not to be bamboozled. Claims for any nutritional supplement are almost always bogus if any of the following apply:

➤ The salesperson creates a nutritional need and then shows how his product fills it.

➤ The product's manufacturers are portrayed as being persecuted by the Food and Drug Administration and other reputable, mainstream providers of nutrition information.

➤ The salesperson says that you're nutritionally deficient without having detailed records of your normal eating habits.

➤ You're told that it will make you lose weight without you having to exercise regularly and consume fewer calories.

Be especially skeptical about products that bear celebrity endorsements. These celebrities are almost always being paid to say what the manufacturers of the products want them to.

Timing Mealtime

Balancing when to eat and when to run can be tough. And that's not just because if you work during normal business hours, then you're probably running when most people are eating breakfast, lunch, or dinner. No, what I'm talking about here is learning how to schedule your runs so that your most recent meal doesn't come back for a second tasting 15 minutes into your run.

This is one of those areas where you're going to have to experiment to find what works best for you. I know some runners who can polish off a lumberjack's breakfast seconds before heading out the door for a morning run and others who swear that they'll have troubled stomachs their entire run if they eat the slightest morsel within several hours of training. There's not much you can do about where you fall on the rockgut scale. When in doubt, err on the side of caution.

Most runners find that they feel much better if they wait at least three hours after their last meal before they run. Running too soon after eating is a big reason that beginners often get side stitches—when you run, your body diverts blood to the exercising parts of your body. You don't want a big meal in your belly demanding to be digested when your heart and legs need all the attention from your circulatory system that they can get.

Footnotes

At a race in Japan once, I startled all the runners near me by popping a potato in my mouth just minutes before the start. I had a few stomach problems during that race, but knew that my opponents were completely psyched out. I won.

On the flip side, there's also great variation among runners concerning how soon they eat after a run. Some runners step in the door and start munching; others don't feel hungry for hours. This amount of time is going to be different even for individual runners from run to run—when it's hot and you finish your run dehydrated and overheated, you're probably not going to be as immediately hungry as on a 50-degree day. The harder you run, the more time you'll probably want to allow before your next meal.

Again, experiment to see what works for you. But here's an important finding from the exercise science labs: If you consume some carbohydrate (it can be in solid or liquid form) within the first 30 minutes of the end of your run, your muscles will absorb those carbohydrates three times as fast as before your run. Although the rate at which they refuel slows some after those first 30 minutes, your muscles remain extra receptive for the first 90 minutes after a run.

What's going on here? Think of your muscles as sponges. Following a run, they're "drier" than at any other time. Just as a dry sponge greedily gobbles water more quickly than a moist sponge, so too do your muscles most want to be refilled when you've just depleted some of their stockpiles.

Why does this absorption matter? Because the gains that you make in your running that allow you to progress occur during the recovery phase following a run. By getting some carbs into your system soon after finishing your run, you therefore speed the recovery process. You'll feel better on your next run, and you'll be better able to nail each of your workouts and progress closer to your goal rate.

Carb refueling is especially important after longer-than-usual runs. Many times, when runners are dragging several hours or even the day after a long run, it's because they waited too long to restock their muscles. As I said, some runners just don't feel like eating any time near after finishing a run. That's OK, but even they would feel better from run to run if they got in the habit of getting a minimal amount of carbs in.

Keep in mind that I'm talking about only 100 to 200 calories in the first hour or so. That's a bagel or a couple of pieces of fruit. If you have a super-sensitive system, liquid carbs are fine (and they'll also help you to get in the important habit of drinking soon after your run). That can mean a sport drink or some diluted fruit juice. Diet sodas don't count because they contain no calories, and therefore, no carbs.

The Least You Need to Know

➤ A good diet will help you to stay healthy enough to run to your ability.

➤ You can't eat your way to becoming a better runner.

➤ The best diet for runners is the same diet that all should people eat.

➤ You should get 60 to 65 percent of your calories from carbohydrates, 15 percent of your calories from protein, and 20 to 25 percent of your calories from fat.

Chapter 14

Crossing the Divide: Cross-Training for Runners

In This Chapter

➤ What is cross-training for runners

➤ Why runners should cross-train

➤ How to blend running with other sports

➤ How to equate cross-training time with running mileage

➤ The best cross-training activities for runners

Tom Fleming, an old marathon rival of mine who is now a coach, asks, "Have you ever seen a Kenyan on a StairMaster? The top runners aren't in the water or biking or using some fancy piece of machinery. They're running." Of course, he's talking about runners who want to compete with the best in the world. But what about you? Should you supplement your running with other aerobic activities? If so, which ones? In this chapter, I'll show you why I think most runners should do some form of cross-training, how to account for your cross-training time, and which cross-training activities are best for runners.

What Is Cross-Training?

Like cooking, *cross-training* is one of those formerly precise terms that has been used in so many ways that it has come to mean pretty much whatever the user wants it to. Just like people call popping a frozen dinner in the microwave cooking, you'll hear people say that they're cross-training when they're mowing their lawn, shoveling snow, or heading out for a night of dancing.

Track Talk
For runners, *cross-training* is using aerobic exercises besides running to supplement your running mileage. It implies planning these activities as an integral part of your program to develop parts of your body that running neglects, as well as to fight injury, burn calories, and boost your aerobic capacity.

Training Tip
When planning activities to supplement your running, don't forget to occasionally include the option of inactivity. Some times, especially on the day after a difficult or long run, your best bet for consolidating the gains from your work is rest rather than more exercise.

I want to use a narrower definition. For the purposes of this chapter, cross-training means aerobic exercises that you plan as part of your regular running program. With this tighter definition, I think that most runners, especially beginners, can benefit from cross-training.

Cross-training doesn't mean anything that you do physically in addition to your running. Household chores, walks around town, and so on should be seen as part of your everyday activities, not as cross-training. Doing yoga or lifting weights doesn't count as cross-training either. Although these stretching and strengthening exercises are important for runners to do (as explained in Chapters 10 and 11), they don't provide the aerobic benefits that cross-training activities do.

Should You Cross-Train?

So what about my old buddy Tom Fleming's point, that if you want to be a good runner, then you should run? After all, you don't become a better cook by washing dishes. First of all, remember that he's talking about runners who are trying to be among the best in the world. These people live by their running mileage, much as a factory lives by the number of widgets it produces per day. (I should know. Having averaged 130 miles per week for most of the '70s and '80s, I was one of these people.)

I'm not suggesting that you replace running with other aerobic activities, but that you supplement your mileage with them. Among the benefits of doing so are the following:

➤ **Fewer muscle imbalances, which are a leading source of injury.** For example, running strengthens and shortens your hamstrings while pretty much neglecting your quadriceps (thigh muscles). But cycling does just the opposite, so combining running with riding helps your legs to keep the proper ratio of strength between front and back muscles.

➤ **Greater aerobic capacity.** A lot of runners can take only so much pounding from running each week before their bodies start to break down. If you find what that level is for you, stay just below it, and add other activities, you can continue to develop your aerobic base beyond what you could just through running. To a large degree, your heart doesn't distinguish what exercise is making it pump more vigorously.

➤ **Greater weight loss.** Because you'll be able to work out more often without getting injured.

➤ **A more interesting exercise routine.** Some people love running so much that they don't need other activities to stay motivated. But a lot of runners find that they look forward to working out more if they alternate among a few sports.

➤ **The chance to work out with non-running friends.** You probably have friends who aren't going to join for a five-mile run, but they might go for an hour's bike ride with you.

Finally, even the most hard-core runners become cross-trainers when they're injured and are desperate to maintain their fitness. If you can run as much as you like without getting injured, can meet your weight goals through running only, are endlessly fascinated by doing just one activity, and regularly do stretching and strengthening exercises that develop whole-body fitness, maybe you don't have to worry about cross-training. If not, read on.

Footnotes

Even some of the best runners in the world have cross-trained to great benefit. In 1980, Alberto Salazar was injured, but he made the U.S. 10K team after running in a pool for most of the months before the Olympic trials. In 1992, Bob Kempainen did a lot of his training on a NordicTrack because he was injured, but he still made the U.S. Olympic Marathon team. Perhaps the oddest cross-training world-class runner was Emil Zatopek, the Czech who won the 5K, 10K, and marathon at the 1952 Olympics. He used to put dirty laundry and sudsy water in a tub and run on the clothes until they were clean.

Cross-Training Time

You wouldn't expect to feel comfortable running if you did it only once a week, but that's the approach that many runners take to their alternative exercises. This approach isn't a good idea, because you'll never become adept enough at the activity for it to contribute significantly toward your fitness. So when you find a second sport that works for you, try to practice it at least twice a week.

Rules of the Road
Ease into new cross-training activities the same way that you progressed gradually as a runner. Don't assume that because you're fit from running, you can take any other sport without risking injury. Learn the basics of motion in your new sport first; when you have the fundamentals down, you can more safely progress.

Unless you're injured and are cross-training as a substitute for running, don't let your aerobic alternatives take precedence over your running. For example, you don't want to put in such a long, hard effort on a bike that your running is compromised for the next few days. Once you get used to your activity, treat it the same as an easy running day. You shouldn't be sore or overly fatigued from your cross-training.

One of the best times to schedule cross-training into your routine is on the day after a hard or long run. The exercise will help to remove waste products that might have built up from the previous day's effort and will help work out any stiffness, but you won't be subjecting tired legs to as much pounding as if you ran.

Comparing Apples and Oranges

One of the reasons that hard-core runners don't do more cross-training is because they don't know how to compare it to their running. The major way that they track their progress is to recite their weekly running mileage to anyone who will listen. A five-mile run is a five-mile run is a five-mile run, so if you only run, keeping records is pretty easy. But what about a two-hour bike ride, a half hour in the pool, or 45 minutes on a stair machine? How do these compare to running miles?

Training Tip
For most cross-training, such as stair machines and hiking, your running shoes will work fine. The exceptions are activities that involve a lot of side-to-side motion, such as tennis or aerobics. In those latter cases, get shoes right for the activity.

My advice is different than what most people are going to tell you. I say, don't worry about it. That's because I'm recommending that you cross-train to *add* to your running, not *replace* it. In that case, there's not much point in obsessing about whether three cycling miles equals one running mile and how many minutes on a rowing machine equal one mile of running. To paraphrase Sigmund Freud, sometimes a two-hour bike ride is just a two-hour bike ride.

Measuring Progress by Effort

If you're cross-training because you're too injured to run, then you want to have some general idea of whether you're doing enough in other sports to compensate for your lack of running. Even when you're cross-training to supplement your running, it's nice to have some general idea of how much work you're doing in a language you're used to. So at the risk of contradicting what I said in the preceding paragraph, try this: Figure that you're getting roughly the same cardiovascular benefits as running for every minute that you cross-train at a similar intensity to the level of effort that you normally sustain while running.

If 4 miles in 40 minutes is an average, medium-effort run for you, then sustaining that level of effort for 40 minutes on a stair machine will provide roughly the same aerobic benefits. Your heart doesn't care what's getting it going, so long as it's an activity that uses major muscle groups for an extended period. Admittedly, this system is imprecise, but I would rather add cross-training to horseshoes and hand grenades and consider "close enough" as being worthwhile than worry too much about exact trade-offs.

After all, those same runners who so precisely say, "I ran 43 miles last week" are deluding themselves unless all of their running is on precisely calibrated courses. Most days, they're making rough estimations about how far they ran based on the amount of time they were out for. I don't see much harm in taking the same approach to cross-training.

However, notice that I said, "every minute that you cross-train at a similar intensity to the level of effort that you normally sustain while running." That's different than just counting the number of minutes that you cross-train. On a stair machine, for example, you'll often spend the first 10 minutes or so getting going; if so, those 10 minutes aren't really at the same intensity as the first 10 minutes of most runs. During a two-hour bike ride, you're likely to spend a nice chunk of that time going downhill, *drafting, coasting,* and so on.

Track Talk
When you run or ride behind someone else doing the same activity, you're *drafting* off of that person. This can save you considerable energy because some of the work you do while exercising on land is pushing your way through the air. In a 5K race on a windy day, drafting can make a given pace as much as 10 percent easier.

Track Talk
When you're on a bike and moving, but not pedaling, you're *coasting*. Because of the ease of coasting, it can be tough to sustain a good workout while cycling. Therefore, you should avoid coasting too much.

If you're new to a sport, it can be difficult to gauge accurately how hard you're working. It might seem as though you're really putting in a good effort, but that could be because your legs are easily tired by the unaccustomed motion, rather than because you're working at a high heart rate. Many runners experience this kind of fatigue on their first few bike rides.

If you have a heart rate monitor, use it when you cross-train to gauge whether your pulse stays in the neighborhood that it usually does when you run. (To learn how to use heart rate monitors, see Chapter 9, "Gadgets on the Go.") Otherwise, expect to spend at least the first few workouts in a new sport learning how to assess your effort.

Choose Your Supplement!

Now that you're convinced cross-training is a good idea, which sport should you pick? The following sections examine the best cross-training options for runners. Keep in mind that in choosing these activities, I'm interested more in what sports best complement running than in which ones provide the best isolated workout.

Track Talk
Nonimpact activities, such as swimming and water running, involve no pounding.

Training Tip
Make convenience the most important factor in deciding which cross-training activities to do. In theory, swimming may be an excellent complement to your running, but not if getting to a pool on a regular basis is a major logistical battle for you.

The Pool Is Cool

If I had to pick one supplementary activity that would help you the most as a runner, it would be swimming. Once you get your stroke down, swimming has many benefits: You can work hard enough to sustain a solid effort; it's a great upper-body strengthener, it's a *nonimpact* activity; and the kicking is terrific for loosening tight tendons and muscles in your feet, ankles, and legs.

The other great use of a pool for runners is water running. This activity is pretty straightforward: You head to the deep end of the pool, usually with a flotation device on, and start running in place. After a few times, it will feel pretty much like running on land. Water running is especially good for injured runners who don't want to lose their land legs during a lay-off, as well as for cross-training runners who get injured beyond a certain level of mileage, but don't like other activities. As with swimming, you have to work a little harder than you would on land to maintain the same heart rate. Many pools now offer water running classes.

The two main drawbacks to swimming are convenience and gauging effort. Finding a suitable pool (one that's big enough to legitimately swim laps in) that isn't too crowded and that has decent hours can be a real challenge. If you don't have good technique, you'll spend your swim flailing around rather than giving your heart a good workout.

Even when you do become adept, comparing swimming to running takes a little extra math. Because you're supported by the water, and because you stay so much cooler than when working out on land, your heart will beat about 15 fewer times per minute for the same effort. So you really have to keep at it to keep your pulse near what it is when you run. Kicking vigorously with your legs is a good way to do this.

Spinning Your Wheels

Cycling has long been a favorite of cross-training runners. Besides the fact that the two exercises complement each other in developing your legs, both give you that great feeling of exercising outside. Cycling can be almost as convenient as running if you don't live in a high-traffic area, and because you cover so much more distance, it's a great way for runners to discover other places to enjoy their favorite sport.

The main drawbacks to cycling are weather and money constraints. As Chapter 16, "Weathering the Elements," explains, you can safely run in just about any conditions. But even the most committed cyclists have to reconsider things during and after heavy rains and snows when they're likely to take a spill. (If you've ever fallen while riding 20 miles per hour, you know that it does a bit more damage than tripping over a root on a run.) Also, once it gets below 30 degrees, cycling outside remains uncomfortable no matter how hard you're working because of the windchill that you generate. It's also not the safest practice to ride in the dark.

Financially, a good bike and the necessary equipment (helmet, gloves, shoes, and so on) can easily cost you close to $1,000. Indoor cycling on a stationary bike involves less hassle and cost, but a lot more boredom. It's tough to be motivated to stay on these machines for long enough to get a real workout in.

If you want to cross-train with cycling, you better be pretty committed to it. Ride at least two days a week so that your legs remain accustomed enough to the activity to allow your heart to reap the benefits.

Rules of the Road
Just like running, all sports have safety rules unique to them. If you're going to spend a lot of time doing a supplementary activity to your running, learn the safety guidelines for that sport.

Training Tip
If there's a piece of exercise equipment that you regularly travel to a gym to use, buying one for your home will help you to work out on it more often if you can afford it.

Rolling with the Changes

I must admit it would take a lot to get me to put on a pair of in-line skates, but that's more because of my love of running and utter lack of coordination than any inherent problem with the activity. Certainly, the ever-growing number of skaters get something out of doing it.

> **Footnotes**
>
> In 1996, more than 10 million Americans in-line skated an average of at least two days per month.

Studies have shown that a similar effort between in-line skating and running requires you to skate twice as fast as you run. As with cycling, it's important to be mindful of your effort. Otherwise, you might find yourself coasting and not getting as good of a workout. But if you stay on top of your effort and have done it enough so that you don't spend all of your time picking yourself off the ground, in-line skating can give you a good workout in a concentrated time, as does running, but without the pounding.

Other Options

The three best remaining aerobic alternatives for runners are cross-country skiing, stair machines, and hiking. Cross-country skiing has been touted as the best all-around exercise because you simultaneously use just about all of your major muscle groups in a non-pounding activity. You and I don't live in Finland, however, so to plan it as a regular part of your program is going to mean hopping on a NordicTrack or similar indoor machine a few times a week. That's a tough routine to sustain for any appreciable amount of time.

Track Talk
An activity that has substantially less pounding than running is considered *low impact*. Such activities include walking and stair climbing.

Stair machines have similar plusses and minuses. They can provide a great workout, assuming you take deep enough steps and don't lean against the rails. They're also *low impact*. But they, too, can require Herculean efforts of will to stay on for at least half an hour a few times a week. That's why most people on them read, listen to music, or watch TV while waiting for the clock to run out.

Hiking offers the great benefit of being outside in beautiful surroundings without the pounding of running. And a mile covered on foot burns roughly the same number of calories whether you run it or walk it. But it's tough enough to find the time to run for short periods a few times a week. For hiking to make sense as part of your regular program, you're going to need at least a block of a couple hours a few times each week.

The Least You Need to Know

➤ Doing another aerobic activity in addition to running will help you to lose weight, stay motivated, and remain injury-free.

➤ Cross-train with a sport that you'll do at least twice a week.

➤ Cross-training should supplement, not replace, your running.

➤ Every minute spent cross-training at an intensity similar to your usual running effort gives roughly the same aerobic benefit as spending that time running.

➤ The best cross-training options for most runners are swimming, cycling, and in-line skating.

Chapter 15

For Women Only

In This Chapter

➤ The few ways that running is different for women than men

➤ Running and the menstrual cycle

➤ Special dietary needs of women runners

➤ Running and the pill

➤ Running before and after pregnancy

As I mentioned in Chapter 1, women have traditionally been discriminated against as much in running as in most other parts of our society. Although a men's marathon was included from the get-go when the modern Olympics began in 1896, a women's marathon wasn't added until 1984. But as I also said in Chapter 1, things are changing for the better for women runners, and for a simple reason: More of them are ignoring the barriers that still exist and are joining the sport. Women in the 20 to 29 age group are among the fastest growing segments in running.

A lot of the old discrimination was blatant sexism. But, as is often the case with discrimination, a lot was based on misunderstanding. Running for women was somehow thought to be different than it is for men. In most cases, it's not. When women start running, they get fitter, just as men do. But there are some female-only running issues, and that's what I'm going to deal with in this chapter, based on what I've learned from talking to women runners, such as Olympic gold medalist Joan Benoit Samuelson and my wife, Gail, as well as from reading.

Are Women Runners Different from Men?

Yes and no. Yes, if you're asking from the standpoint of "Can they run as fast?" But, more importantly, no, if you mean, "Does running affect women differently?"

> **Footnotes**
>
> The Boston Marathon didn't officially allow women to enter the race until 1972. To enter that year, women had to meet the same qualifying standard then in place for men, 3:30. Eight women ran, led by Nina Kuscsik in 3:10:26.

If the two are equally well-trained, the average woman is going to be slower than the average man, from the 100-meter dash on up to the marathon. Women have certain disadvantages when they compete against men:

➤ Women have smaller hearts than men, so the heart pumps less blood with each beat. To run a given pace, a woman's heart rate has to be higher than a man's.

➤ Women have lower *hemoglobin* levels than men, so less oxygen is sent to working muscles.

➤ Women have higher essential body fat stores than men.

➤ Women's lower levels of testosterone mean that women have less muscle mass than men.

Track Talk
Hemoglobin is a protein in red blood cells that carries oxygen from your lungs to your muscles. With less hemoglobin, women have less oxygen per unit of blood.

Working together, these unavoidable physical factors make women, on average, 10 to 12 percent slower than men at all commonly run distances.

So, on the whole, women are always going to be slower than men. I suppose it's easy for me to say this, but I wouldn't make that big a deal out of it. Although women are not as fast as men, running has the same effect on both genders. Women have traditionally been discouraged from running as much or as hard as men, but there's no basis for this practice. Studies have consistently shown that women who train at the same level as men see the same amount of increase in their fitness.

Footnotes

Title IX, which banned gender discrimination in federally funded high school and college sports, was signed into law in 1972. Since then, women's participation in all sports, including running, has skyrocketed.

Remember that strange phrase, VO_2 max, from Chapter 2? It's your body's ability to use oxygen while working and is the most important measure of your cardiovascular fitness. Six months to a year after starting to run, previously sedentary people can expect their VO_2 max values to increase by 20 to 30 percent. That's equally true for women and men.

What you probably care about a whole lot more than maximum speed is your running—how to get fitter, how to find the time for it, how to stick with it, and so on. The answers to those questions are the same for all runners. That's not to say that women runners aren't going to want answers to questions that we men never to have to think about. The following sections examine some of the most common areas of concern.

Footnotes

The women's world record for the marathon is 2:21:06, by Norway's Ingrid Kristiansen. In 1996, only 40 American men ran faster for the distance.

Running and the Menstrual Cycle

Just as the effects of menstruation itself differ greatly from woman to woman, the effects of menstruation on running performance vary greatly as well. Some women notice no difference in performance; others notice a great deal of difference.

If your period is going to affect your running, it's most likely to occur during the premenstrual and early flow phases of the cycle. The good news is that many women runners find that their running helps to ease cramps, bloating, headaches, fatigue, and all of those other friendly monthly visitors. To best deal with the effects of menstruation, track how your cycle affects your running in a training log, and then plan accordingly. For example, if you notice that running often

Training Tip
Be sure to drink a lot of water if you have bloating during your premenstrual phase. You might think that drinking water will only make you more bloated, but that bloating is caused by sodium retention. Drinking enough water will flush that sodium out of your system and will help you to feel better on your runs.

seems harder during your premenstrual phase, accept that and don't try runs that are longer or harder than usual during this time.

On the not-so-good side, running can lead to increased bleeding. Some of the painkillers, such as ibuprofen, that help with other side effects can also reduce bleeding. The increased bleeding usually isn't so great that it's visible. But if you're worried about this, do what Olympic gold medalist in the marathon, Joan Benoit Samuelson, does and run with a tampon in a plastic bag pinned inside of your shorts or tights.

Track Talk
Amenorrhea is the absence of regular menstrual cycles. The main cause seems to be not eating enough to meet your energy needs. It can lead to weakened bones and should be avoided.

Women runners sometimes don't have periods. This condition is called *amenorrhea*, and although it might sound like a dream come true, it's not good. It usually means that little or no estrogen is circulating in your body, which can lead to your bones becoming weaker, as well as short-term infertility.

The causes are complex, but most experts think that amenorrhea is caused more often by not eating enough than by exercising too much. Running alone can't be named as the cause, given that some women train more than 100 miles a week and still have regular periods. If your periods stop or become irregular (more often than every 25 days or less frequent than every 35 days), see a doctor. Just don't let him or her convince you that running is solely to blame.

Women of Steel: Iron Needs

Women runners should be more careful than men runners about preventing low iron stores. Iron is used to produce hemoglobin in your red blood cells. As mentioned before, one of the reasons that women are, on average, slower than men is because women have less hemoglobin. This condition is made worse if your iron stores are low, because then your hemoglobin levels become lower. When hemoglobin levels decrease, less oxygen reaches your muscles when you run, so running your normal pace feels harder.

Why are women runners more susceptible to low iron stores? For starters, all women lose iron through menstrual blood. On top of that, women runners tend to be more careful about their diet than sedentary women. That's usually good, except that one of the things that women runners often get more selective about is eating meat. Limiting meat can be a good way to cut fat out of your diet, but it also can mean too severely limiting your iron-rich food choices.

Good food sources of iron that aren't high in fat include the following:

➤ Lean red meat and dark poultry

➤ Dark green, leafy vegetables

➤ Legumes

➤ Dried fruit

➤ Whole-grain or enriched cereals and bread

You can increase how much iron you absorb from a food by eating foods rich in vitamin C at the same time. Using cast-iron cookware also helps. On the other hand, you decrease how much iron you absorb from foods when you drink coffee or tea with meals. Premenopausal women runners should shoot for an iron intake of at least 15 milligrams (mg) per day; post-menopausal women need 10.

Other reasons that women runners might have low iron stores apply to men, too: loss through sweat and urine, increased blood volume with training (which lowers iron concentration in the blood), and what's known as footstrike hemolysis, which is the breakdown of red blood cells from your feet repeatedly hitting the ground. When you have blood tests done, ask for your hemoglobin and serum ferritin (a measure of your body's iron stores) levels to be checked. Normal hemoglobin concentration for women is from 12 to 16 grams per 100 milliliters of blood. Because of the increased blood volume that comes with running, a reading of 11 can be considered safe for a women runner, but anything below that is asking for trouble. The acceptable range for serum ferritin is 10 to 200 milligrams per milliliter of blood. Some experts caution that any reading below 25 can hurt your running.

Training Tip
You'll absorb three times as much iron from a breakfast of cereal and toast if you drink orange juice rather than coffee with it.

Running and Birth Control

Obviously, birth control is an incredibly personal choice. I just want to tell you what some women runners have experienced. A few studies have found that women runners are less likely than sedentary women to take birth control pills. Many women report that they just don't feel as good while running when they're on the pill. Fatigue and nausea are common side effects of being on the pill, as is weight gain.

Because the pill eliminates the premenstrual and early flow phases of a period, the pill can be a good birth control choice for women runners who feel that their running suffers at these times. Overall, though, most women runners who have found a successful alternative to the pill prefer to avoid oral contraceptives.

Two for the Road: Running and Pregnancy

In June 1995, while 8 1/2 months pregnant, Sue Olsen ran a marathon in 4:00:50. The following week, Olsen competed in a 24-hour race. Less than 30 hours after finishing that mega long event, she gave birth to a healthy son who weighed seven pounds, three ounces. OK, so Olsen is a bit on the extreme side. But I thought you should know about her because she, and her healthy son, are evidence that being pregnant doesn't necessarily mean lying on your back for nine months eating chocolate-covered pickles.

Play, Don't Labor: Running While Pregnant

Pregnant women used to be told any exercise beyond even the most low-key, minimal exertion would endanger both their health and that of their fetus. The main concern was that the mother and fetus wouldn't gain enough weight to produce a healthy baby come birth. It was also thought that when a pregnant woman runs, the fetus would be harmed because of less oxygen and blood flow going to the uterus.

Because of fears like these, the American College of Obstetrics and Gynecology (ACOG) used to say that pregnant women shouldn't work out strenuously for more than 15 minutes and that they should keep their heart rates below 140 beats per minute. In other words, don't really run. A lot of faithful women runners chose to ignore those recommendations when they became pregnant. As they did, and seemed to produce normal, healthy babies, more studies were done about running and pregnancy.

Among other good things, these studies found that the fears of damage to the fetus by running moms-to-be were unfounded. The pregnant body has compensatory mechanisms for decreased oxygen and blood flow to the uterus. It's been shown that both the woman and fetus have all the fuel they need when the woman runs, even in the late stages of pregnancy, when fetal growth really takes off. Hey, Sue Olsen had to get energy somewhere during that 24-hour race, after all.

In terms of birth and after, studies have shown no real difference between sedentary pregnant women and active ones in these important matters:

➤ Complications of pregnancy, labor, and delivery

➤ Type of delivery (C-section versus vaginal)

➤ Circumference of the baby's head

➤ Overall health of the baby

➤ Weight of the baby at birth

As for weight gain during pregnancy, one study found that active pregnant women put on about 30 pounds each, compared to 39 to 42 pounds for nonexercisers. ACOG recommends that most women gain 25 to 35 pounds.

One study compared women who worked out vigorously, including running, to those whose only exercise while pregnant was walking. When the children of these women were five years old, those of the intense exercisers scored higher on tests of intelligence, coordination, and language skills.

Because of all of this evidence that vigorous exercise is safe, ACOG revised its guidelines in 1994. Now, it encourages women who are fit and active when they become pregnant to remain so as long as they can comfortably during pregnancy. So long as you keep in close contact with your doctor and use common sense, ACOG says, it's OK to run vigorously throughout your entire pregnancy.

Now, whether Sue Olsen's exploits would get the ACOG seal of approval, I'm not sure. But I bet they wouldn't have any problem with Joan Benoit Samuelson, who ran five miles on the morning before she gave birth to her second child, and remembers the run as one of the favorites of her whole life. Remember, this is a woman who won the Olympic Marathon!

Sue and Joan are among the luckiest ones. No matter how many green lights ACOG gives you, and no matter how dedicated you are, there comes a time when intensive weight-bearing exercise like running becomes too uncomfortable to be worth doing for most pregnant women. If and when that occurs will vary from woman to woman and even from pregnancy to pregnancy for repeat moms. That's where the common sense part of ACOG's current guidelines come into play.

When running isn't an option anymore, many women runners turn to less-intensive cross-training options. When Janis Klecker, a 1992 Olympian in the marathon, was six months into her second pregnancy and pregnant with twins, running became a hindrance rather than a help. So she switched to swimming, walking, and riding a stationary bike. An Olympic teammate of hers from 1992, Gwyn Coogan, ran until the seventh month of her pregnancy, and then switched to hiking, biking, and swimming. The key is that they sensed when the running wasn't worth doing anymore, accepted that temporary situation, and found other, more comfortable, ways to stay fit and active.

Rules of the Road
Although the latest thinking encourages pregnant women to exercise vigorously, it's still important not to overdo it. Your body temperature shouldn't get above 101 degrees while running when you're pregnant.

Training Tip
When you're pregnant, don't compare your running to your pre-pregnant days. If you go to races, forget your usual goals and just participate to have fun.

Post-Partum Expression

The answer to how much and how fast to run after giving birth, just like how much and how fast to run before giving birth, differs from woman to woman. A lot of it has to do with how tough your pregnancy and delivery were. A standard guideline is to wait about six weeks after a vaginal delivery, a bit more for a C-section. Again, though, those are just general guidelines. Part of being a runner is being in touch with your body, and you should have a feel for when it's right to get going again. Gwyn Coogan started running again only 10 days after giving birth, but Janis Klecker waited eight weeks.

Footnotes

Some women return to running after pregnancy with few problems. In 1991, Britain's Liz McColgan placed third in the world cross-country championships, just four months after giving birth!

As some women runners have pointed out, you never know until it's too late if you tried to come back too soon. In this sense, starting to run again after giving birth can be a lot like starting again after an injury. You're always going to be wondering if it's OK to try to progress, and you're going to feel a lot different running than you used to. That's especially the case for new mothers who are probably trying to run with more weight than they had before being pregnant.

Your joints and ligaments remain loose for about nine months to a year after delivery. This looseness makes you especially susceptible to injury during this time, so you should avoid hills and uneven terrain. Put all those factors together, and most women runners who have been through the process, even highly motivated ones like Coogan and Klecker, think it's a good idea to err on the side of caution.

Some women say that once they return to their regular running program after giving birth, they feel much stronger. Of course, there's a psychological side to this. As Louise Kelley, a top local runner in the Washington, DC area, says about being a running mother, there's nothing like a forced nine months off to get you really motivated.

The Least You Need to Know

➤ In terms of the effects of training, women runners are no different than men.

➤ The average women is slower than the average man because of physical differences.

➤ Although a great variation among women exists, most women runners find that running helps during their menstrual cycle.

➤ Women runners should consume more iron-rich foods than sedentary women.

Chapter 16

Weathering the Elements

In This Chapter

➤ Why it's harder to run in heat and humidity

➤ How to run safely in hot weather

➤ Why winter running is better than you think

➤ When the weather is too bad to run

➤ Skin care for runners

I've run through more than 30 New England winters. I've run in Arizona in the spring, in New York and Ohio in the fall, and even run a marathon in Vietnam in the summer. Let's just say I get around.

So I always laugh a little when, on a slightly cloudy day, someone asks me, "You're not going to run *today*, are you?" People ask this because in our society, most inactive people have no real exposure to the elements—they're almost always in a house, a car, or an office. Running regularly gets you outside. In fact, finding a certain beauty in all kinds of weather, and living in harmony with Mother Nature, is one of the great appeals of running.

I'm not going to lie to you and say that I always love running in all kinds of weather. You have to respect the conditions and plan accordingly, or it can get pretty frightful, rather than delightful, out there. Once you learn how to do that, though, you'll be good to go pretty much anytime, anywhere. You'll see autumn sunsets, winter wildlife, summer showers, and spring blossoms in ways that most people never do. In this chapter, I'll explain how to cope with some of the more extreme weather conditions that you'll face as you stick with a year-round running program.

A Hot Time in the City

You know that you tire more quickly when it's 90 degrees rather than 50 degrees, even if you're just taking a leisurely stroll. And you know that the harder you work, the more tired heat makes you. But why is that? And what can you do about it?

When you run in the heat, your body sends more blood to your skin to cool you via evaporation. As a result, less blood, which carries oxygen, goes to your leg muscles, and they have to work harder just to maintain your usual pace. Also, the warmer it is, the more you sweat. This is good, because sweating helps to cool you as your perspiration evaporates. But it's also bad, because your blood volume decreases. With less blood returning to your heart, your heart has to pump more often to keep the same amount of blood circulating throughout your body. And when your heart rate increases, you're working harder.

Footnotes

Even the best runners in the world slow significantly in the heat. At the 1976 Boston Marathon, where the temperature reached 101 degrees, Jack Fultz won in 2:20:19. This is the slowest winning time there since 1968. Two years later, when it was 47 degrees at the start, Fultz ran 2:11:17. (I won.)

Running is even tougher on humid days. You generate all that sweat, and it's supposed to cool you down, but the air is so moist that it can't absorb much more water. So your sweat stays on your skin rather than evaporating, and your body just keeps producing more and more sweat, and you just keep getting more and more tired. That's why it's a lot tougher to run on a 90-degree day in the humid Northeast part of the country, like Washington, DC, than in someplace like New Mexico. Out in the desert, it's hot, but dry, and your sweat can cool you like it's supposed to.

The Dangers of Dehydration

The upshot of all this dripping sweat is a dropping pace. One study found that for each one percent of body weight that you lose because of *dehydration*, your running performance falls by three percent. Bear in mind that one percent of body weight isn't much—if you weigh 150 pounds, that's only 1.5 pounds, or 24 ounces. It's not unusual to lose three or four pounds of water in an hour of running on a hot day. This loss causes your performance to sag by more than five percent, which can be as much as a minute slower per mile. Are you starting to see why it's so tough to feel comfortable while running in the heat?

You also need to consider cumulative dehydration. Cumulative dehydration is what happens when it's hot for several days in a row, and you don't replace all the fluid you lost after each run. Suppose that during a hot week, an 150-pound runner doesn't rehydrate himself completely each day. By the end of the week, he has a cumulative loss of two pounds of water—that's more than one percent of his weight. As a result, his performance is off by more than three percent by week's end, but he may not make the connection to dehydration. A lot of runners, myself included most summers, go through the hottest parts of the year chronically dehydrated. As a result, our running suffers.

Rules of the Road
If you feel dizzy while running in the heat, stop, get out of the sun, and drink water. You're probably suffering from heat exhaustion. If you stop sweating, stop running immediately. You're probably suffering from the more serious heat stroke. This condition requires immediate medical attention.

Beating the Heat

Now that I've completely turned you off on running in the heat, what can you do to fight dehydration? Drink, drink, then drink some more. Your thirst mechanism is imperfect; by the time you're thirsty, you're dehydrated.

How do you know if you're staying on top of staying hydrated? First, weigh yourself before and after runs in hot weather. However much lighter you are at the end of the run, drink at least that amount of water within the first two hours of your run. Remember, a pint's a pound the world around, so for every pound you lost on the run, drink 16 ounces.

Rules of the Road
Besides weighing yourself before and after runs, watch your urine during the day. It should always be clear in color and frequent. If it's dark or infrequent, you need to drink more water, even if you're not thirsty.

Don't cheat on this method if one of the reasons you're running is to lose weight. The weight that you lose on a run in the heat isn't fat. It's water and needs to be replaced if you want to keep running. Your blood and other body fluids help to remove waste products and to carry nutrients to muscle tissues, so the faster you replace lost fluids, the more quickly you'll recover from run to run. Replacing water doesn't have anything to do with how many calories you burn on a run, which is what counts in determining how much fat you lose. If anything, quickly replacing water weight loss will *help* you lose weight because you'll feel better from day to day, and you'll be more likely to stick with your running in tough conditions.

For some reason, it's tough for most people to stay hydrated. Maybe that's because eating is one of life's great joys, but after awhile, drinking water just gets boring. Make it easy to drink water often throughout the day. One coach I know tells his runners to keep a two-liter bottle of water at their desks at work. They're supposed to finish it at least once from when they get to the office until they go home. I also know runners who are in the habit of stopping for a drink at every water fountain they pass during the day, regardless of whether they're thirsty. It's also a good idea to keep a bottle of water by your bed. I know this sounds like a lot of work, maybe even borderline obsessive. But it's worth it, because you'll feel so much better on your runs.

Training Tip

Most people can absorb only about seven ounces of fluid every 15 minutes. That's why it's better to drink small amounts of water throughout the day and during your runs instead of drinking a lot at once.

Not only is it important to drink water before, after, and between runs, it's important to drink during them as well. I keep a water bottle hidden in the woods a few miles from my house. When I run by it, I stop and drink, and then restash it. When it's empty, I carry it home, refill it, and drive it back to its hiding spot. Here are other ways to conveniently get drinks on the run:

Training Tip

On really hot days, it feels great to pour water over your head. But doing so doesn't fight dehydration. Pour that water down your throat, where it can do you some good.

➤ Plan your route so that you'll pass schools, gas stations, and other places that have water fountains.

➤ Plan your route so that you pass your home once or twice. Have a water bottle waiting for you at the end of driveway.

➤ The night or morning before a longer run, drive over your route, stashing bottles along the way.

➤ On the hottest days, carry water with you. Many runners prefer fannypacks that hold bottles to keep their hands free and their arm action normal.

If you can use some of these methods to make sure you get some fluid every 15 to 20 minutes during your run, you'll last a lot longer in the heat. I also like to drink two or three glasses of water a few minutes before I run. Sometimes the water sloshes around in my stomach at the start, but I know it will help me by the end of the run.

Nothing beats water for pure hydration. But you're more likely to drink enough if you enjoy a variety of fluids. What are other good options for just before, during, and right after a run? Studies have shown that sport drinks that are four to eight percent carbohydrate, like most of the commercially available ones, are absorbed as quickly as water. They have the added plus of providing energy. Fruit juices aren't absorbed as quickly; dilute them by half with water. Carbonated beverages aren't a great idea because they might upset your stomach and because they make you feel full. If you drink a carbonated drink, you might think that you're more hydrated than you are.

Finally, when you run can make a big difference in how much the heat takes out of you especially when you're not *acclimatized* (used to running in the heat). Avoid the hottest times of the day. This is one instance where you're at an advantage if you have to squeeze in your run before or after work. Still, be careful: The humidity is highest in the morning, and it can still be pretty oppressive at 7 p.m. in some places in the summer. When in doubt, slow your pace from the start, rather than having your dehydrated body slow it for you near the end.

> **Training Tip**
> If you drink caffeinated drinks or alcohol, drink at least an equal amount of extra water for each drink to balance the dehydrating effect. For example, if you have two beers with dinner, drink at least an extra 24 ounces of water.

> **Track Talk**
> *Acclimatization* is the process of becoming used to running in the heat. Most runners need at least a week of shorter, easier workouts in hotter weather before they feel ready to resume their normal training routine.

The Winter Wonderland

One of the main reasons that running in the winter can be so nice is because running in the summer can be so tough. With all the heat that you generate after a few minutes of running, you can be warmer running outside in 40-degree weather than inside your 68-degree home. So you stay warm enough to stay comfortable, but don't get so hot that you get really dehydrated. The best of both worlds!

> **Footnotes**
> Thanks to all the high-tech gear, it's a lot easier to be a comfortable winter runner than even 20 years ago. Before tights were invented, runners trained through the cold months in heavy cotton sweats or long johns. In 1973, I ran a 20-mile race in blue jeans.

You can't get away with running in just anything in the winter. As explained in Chapter 8, "From Top to Bottom: The Right Running Apparel," some necessary items of clothing

Rules of the Road
When running, you generate up to 11 times the amount of heat that you do when at rest. If you're warm at the start of a cold-weather run, you're going to be too hot later on. Dress for how warm you'll be 10 minutes into your run.

Track Talk
Windchill is usually described incorrectly. Regardless of what they tell you on TV, it's not how cold it feels when you combine the temperature and wind velocity. Rather, it's how quickly the cold and wind make you lose body heat. For runners, who create a lot of heat even in the wintriest conditions, the windchill is only of concern when it's so low that you're at risk of frostbite.

will help you stay comfortable when it's cold. The key is wearing the right gear for the right conditions, which usually involves layering. For more on that concept, see Chapter 8.

The Freeze-Your-Lungs Myth

Except for the few hottest days of the year, most people aren't going to question your sanity when you're out running in July or August. But keep running through the winter, and eventually someone is going to ask you, "Aren't you afraid that you'll freeze your lungs?"

Even my dad used to ask me this when I started running in high school. I was taught to respect my elders, so I didn't laugh in his face or anything, but this question is one of the silliest I've ever heard. Have you ever met someone who has frozen a lung? Of course not. As the air you breathe works its way into your lungs, it's warmed more than enough to keep it from freezing anything.

I bet you have met someone who was in pretty good shape, but stopped working out when it got cold, and started the spring with more weight and less fitness. That's a shame, and an unnecessary one, because winter running can be some of the best of the year. And I'm a New Englander, so it's not like I'm sitting here espousing the joys of winter running from my house in Los Angeles.

I get a certain pride out of knowing that on those short, dark, cold days with plenty of *windchill*, when most people are always under shelter, I've been outside moving under my own power. I know that when people look out their windows and see me running down their street they think that I'm both miserable and insane. Those people don't know that when I'm done with my run, I'll enjoy being inside that much more.

Running in the winter involves a bigger mental aspect to it than running during the rest of the year. I admit that after doing this for 30 years, I still sometimes have a tough time getting psyched to run when there's only been eight hours of daylight for the last couple of months. You just need to keep focused on your goals. After awhile, you'll learn how to get out the door and through those tough first few minutes until you start getting warmed up. I can usually do this by reminding myself how much better I'll feel after my run. Also, ask yourself if you would be so ready to bag your run if it were sunny and 70 degrees.

Footing, Short Days, and Icy Roads

The lack of light, not the potential freezing of your lungs, is the biggest threat to your well-being when you run in the winter. Watch your footing. Try to run on level surfaces that you're familiar with and choose the most well-lit routes. Be extra careful after snow or ice storms. Snow on the ground can often help your night vision, because it reflects what light there is. But under that snow may be patches of ice.

Also, watch traffic even more than you usually do. Don't assume that cars can see you or that, if they do, they can get out of the way quickly. Just as snow and ice can make you slip around during your runs, they also can cause cars to careen out of control. Fortunately, most good winter running apparel made these days has reflective features. If yours doesn't, you can buy reflective strips and a reflective vest at most running stores. Almost all good running shoes have reflective elements built into their design. These elements are a must if you want to run safely in the dark.

Neither Sleet, nor Hail: Foul-Weather Running

Along with the frozen-lung query, one of the other most common weather-related questions I hear is, "What do you do when it rains?" The answer: Get wet. What I mean, without being too much of a martyr about it, is that part of being a runner is coping with the hand that Mother Nature deals. Again, most people in our society have lost their connection to the outdoors. The only running in the rain they can imagine is from their office building to the car so that they don't get wet.

But what do you do after a run? You get in the shower; you get wet. Why is so horrible to get wet *during* your run? Unless the rain is cold, running in the rain can be incredibly enjoyable. Think about when you were a kid and how you splashed in puddles or how good it felt to be in the rain in the middle of summer.

Of course, running in the rain isn't always ideal. As I said, a cold rain is not that fun. You have to be extra careful, especially if you're running near a lot of traffic. Cars aren't going to be able to see you as well. But most times, putting on the right gear (see Chapter 8) and a baseball or painter's cap is the only added step you need to take to have a great run. When you get home, just be sure to change into dry clothes as soon as possible.

Training Tip
On windy days, plan your route so that the wind is primarily at your back on the way home. You don't want to build up a bit of a sweat, and then get too cold when you're facing a headwind on the return trip. It's also not much fun to fight a headwind when you're tired toward the end of your run.

Rules of the Road
When running after a snowstorm, wear darker clothing so that drivers can see you better against the white backdrop. If you have more than one pair of running shoes, wear the one with the most studded outsole so that you'll have better traction.

Notice how I keep mentioning cold rain? I'm not going to tell you that being a runner means you stick to your planned run no matter what the conditions. Freezing rain, sleet, hail—when the weather is that bad, it's usually time to reconsider. Shorten your run, sticking close to home so that you can end the run quickly if conditions deteriorate. Or, if the nasty stuff is only going to be around for a day, don't feel guilty about taking the day off. You can get battered around if you always try to run in those conditions. I once had to take cover while running during a major hail storm in Arizona.

The only other weather I really fear is lightning. I just don't go out when it's striking. Fortunately, you can usually wait for it to pass and get in a nice post-storm run.

Made in the Shade: Sun Protection

People used to think that a great tan was one of running's main side benefits. Now we know better. There are almost a million new cases of skin cancer every year in the United States. My grandfather died from a melanoma, and my mom has had skin cancer, so I'm especially aware of this problem. But it's not just those of us with a family history of these problems who need to be careful, especially with the growing hole in the ozone layer. These days, smart runners can take a few, easy steps to lower their risk of overexposure to the sun.

Rules of the Road
A hat provides good sun protection, but can also trap a lot of heat on warm, sunny days. To keep the sun off of your face, but also stay cool, wear a visor.

The major one is to wear a waterproof sunscreen. It should have an SPF (sun protection factor) rating of at least 15. Ten to 15 minutes before your run, apply it liberally to any body parts that are going to be exposed. In the past, you may have heard that these sport sunscreens interfered with sweating, making you much hotter. Recent research, however, has shown that you'll sweat just as much when you wear sunscreen, so glop it on.

Other steps to lower your sun exposure while running include the following:

➤ Wear something on your head to shield your face.

➤ Wear sport sunglasses to protect your eyes.

➤ Try not to run when the sun is strongest, from 10 a.m. to 2 p.m.

➤ Run in the shade. (You'll also stay cooler if you do.)

If you're lucky enough to be running during daylight hours in the winter, don't forget the sunscreen. The sun isn't as strong then, but it can do its work nonetheless, especially when it's reflecting off snow.

The Least You Need to Know

➤ For every one percent of your body weight that you lose to dehydration, your running performance suffers by three percent.

➤ If you're thirsty, you're already dehydrated.

➤ The best way to prevent dehydration is to drink small amounts of water throughout the day, rather than a few big drinks all at once.

➤ If you have the right gear, the winter can be one of the best times of the year to run.

➤ To prevent skin cancer, wear sunscreen with an SPF of at least 15 when you run.

Part 4
Join the Human Race

This part is about going to races. I've always been a racer, from my first race in 1963, to my last four Boston Marathon victories in 1980, up to today, when I'm in my 50s. Racing is the icing on the running cake, and it's sweeter than any dessert I've ever had.

Find out why so many runners race, and where they go to do it. You'll experience basic workouts that will improve your running, even if you decide never to attend a race. Then I'll detail more specific training for the most popular race distances, from 5K to the marathon. To top it all off, I've included a list of my 10 favorite races from the thousand or so that I've run in my life.

Chapter 17

The Finish Line: Why You Should Race

In This Chapter

➤ Why runners attend races

➤ How racing for time helps to keep you motivated

➤ How people help others by running marathons

➤ Why separate age groups for older runners are good

More than 15,000 running races are held in the United States every year. This chapter explores some of the main reasons that people like to go to races. Most of those reasons might not be what you think, and they don't all involve killing yourself to shave one second from your 5K time.

People Pay to Do This?

The average road race is held early on a Sunday morning. A standard road race with T-shirts, awards, post-race refreshments, and so on costs $15 to $25 to enter. In other words, most people running in them have gone to bed early on a Saturday night, gotten up at least as early on a Sunday morning as on a regular workday, and then handed over the cost of a nice dinner for the opportunity to inflict pain on themselves. Sounds like they're the idiots, huh?

They're far from it, and I'm not just sensitive to that charge because I go to 25 to 30 races a year. At some level, these runners realize that far from being masochists, they're indulging themselves. That's right—indulging themselves! Racing is the proverbial icing on the running cake.

Your regular training gives you the big health and fitness benefits that are the most important thing about running for most people, but experiencing only that part of running can get a little tedious. You need some excitement and some variety in anything that you do regularly, no matter how much you love it. In running, that excitement and variety most often comes from going to a race. You don't even have to try to run harder than you do when you run on your own. There's just something about lining up with your fellow runners and experiencing the same course together that adds an element to your running that's impossible to find otherwise.

Footnotes

How's this for a reason to race? Fermin Cacho of Spain won the gold medal at 1500 meters in the 1992 Olympics after the king of Spain promised him $1 million for a victory.

Say you really like to cook. Which would you rather do: Always cook for just you and your spouse, making pretty much the same types of dishes at the same time of day? Or would you rather use those daily cooking sessions as the main way to enjoy your hobby, but also throw a dinner party once in a while where you get to put it all on the line and let yourself and others see just what you're capable of? Most people would choose the second option, and that's why you see so many people at races.

Let's continue that dinner party analogy just a bit farther. Say you invite a few friends over for dinner. You don't worry about how your culinary skills compare to Wolfgang Puck's, do you? No. You do the best you can given your background and ability, and afterward you're rewarded with the feeling of a job well done.

Rules of the Road
For races up to 10K (6.2 miles), your weekly mileage should be at least three times the distance that you want to race. For example, you should be running at least 15 miles a week before attempting a five-mile race.

The same is true of nearly all of the people in any race. They know that they don't have to look like Frank Shorter or Joan Benoit Samuelson to race. They know that races give their running a focus and are a great source of motivation for getting out the door most days. Preparing for a race that's a few months away is one of the best examples of setting the challenging, specific goals that were discussed in Chapter 6.

Many beginning runners have a sense that their running would be more exciting if they went to races, but they're afraid that they'll finish last and be embarrassed. As Richard

Nixon would have said, let me say this about that: First, most races have at least a few hundred runners in them. Just like only one person is going to finish first, only one person is going to finish last. The odds of that being you are pretty long, believe me.

More important, if it is you, so what? No one has ever been shot or even booed for finishing last in a road race. In fact, some of the loudest applause from spectators in races are for those near the back of the pack. The spectators recognize the extra effort that these runners are putting out. Adding to that applause are often many of the runners who have finished their races, and then hung around the finish area to cheer on their fellow runners. That kind of camaraderie with your fellow runners is one of the main draws that races have.

Racing's Best-Kept Secret: It's Fun!

People who haven't been to races aren't going to know this, so you'll just have to take my word for it until you see it for yourself: You'd be hard-pressed to find an event more filled with smiles and unambiguous goodwill than your local road race. Put another way, why should you race? Because it's fun!

A road race is the closest thing to a mobile party that I can think of. (Well, the closest legal thing.) Everywhere you look, there are smiles, cheers, laughs, and heartfelt congratulations from one runner to another. There's music before and after (sometimes even during), there's great food after, prizes are given out, and kids are roaming all around—sounds more like a circus than someplace where a bunch of skinny masochists gather to be miserable together, doesn't it?

Of course, most people aren't laughing it up and smiling during the race; they're working pretty darned hard. But that effort explains the festive atmosphere afterward. The runners have pushed and challenged themselves, and now they're all celebrating the sense of accomplishment that doing so brings.

In life, isn't one extreme of something usually more enjoyable if you've recently been near the other extreme? Isn't a sunny day more special when it's been raining for a week than when it's the 10th bright day in a row? Doesn't your easy chair feel best when you've been working your hardest? That's why races are so much fun. Once you've experienced a race, you'll agree with me that there's a certain kind of fun that comes from challenging yourself within sharply defined parameters while others around you are doing the same.

Training Tip
After a race, talk to the people who finished near you. These people are good potential training partners because you're currently at roughly the same level of ability as they are.

Personal Bests

I've always been a competitor, ever since I was the fastest kid in a run during gym class in school. Seeing how fast I can run has long been my primary motivation to be a runner. Oddly enough, that's why I stopped running for a few years after college. My goal then had been to break 9:00 for two miles, and I did. I didn't see the point in racing anymore, so I didn't see the point in running anymore. (Now, of course, I know better. What's that about youth being wasted on the young?)

I was fortunate to be able to win races when I was younger. I'm not going to lie to you and tell you that doing so wasn't incredibly satisfying. Let me tell you, if you ever need motivation to get out the door for a run on a tough New England winter day, try telling yourself that you'll be defending your title at the Boston Marathon in a couple of months. It worked wonders for me.

But even when I raced for place, I was also always focused on my finishing times in races. Now that I don't win races anymore, I'm even more fanatical about them. I'm certainly not alone in that regard. For many runners, setting personal records, or getting under a certain barrier for a distance, or seeing how their time at a race this year compares to what they ran there last year, or any of the million other ways that you can look at your running times provides the biggest reason to race. There's something intoxicating about racing against yourself.

Your race times provide an objective record of your accomplishment on that day. There's just no way around it—your race time is how long it took you to run this course on this day. Unlike other sports competitions, races are about unadulterated human performance. In other sports, you're maneuvering against your opponents and trying to finesse some piece of equipment. When you race for time, it's just you, the elements, and the clock.

Footnotes

I ran my first organized race in 1963. It was a five-lap-to-the-mile race put on by the Connecticut Parks and Recreation Department as part of its summer games program when I was in high school. I won in 5:20.

Nothing else I've found in sports gives you that yes-or-no sense of accomplishment that racing for time does. Suppose you play on a softball team. How do you know whether you've had a good game? There are so many variables that you don't have primary control over. Did you get two hits because you swung the bat well or because the other team's pitcher stunk? What about when you made that nice play at third base, but the first baseman flubbed your throw, or the umpire made the wrong call? There's none of that uncertainty when you race for time.

Earlier in this chapter, I told you how aiming for a race is one of the best ways to set the short-term goals I keep recommending. On top of that, aiming toward a race and having a time goal for it helps to keep you running even more. It lends a logic to your training—with the race as your goal, you have a better idea of what types of running you should be doing. Those time goals are a great answer for that little voice in your head that's occasionally going to say, "Why are you doing this?"

Charitable Contributions

Races have long been venues for raising money for charities. I've always liked being able to tie in doing something good for myself with helping others. Chapter 23 details some of my favorite charity runs. Most of the people running these kinds of races would probably have participated in them anyway; the money raised for charity is a nice side consequence of them doing so.

However, one of the biggest trends in American racing is charity running that works the other way around—people enter races (usually marathons) solely for the purpose of raising money for charity. This approach has long been applied to other activities. For example, think of the AIDS Walks or the March of Dimes. The new charity running emphasis at races is much the same, except that the runners use races that already exist, rather than events that are created specifically for them.

The biggest of these types of programs is called Team in Training, run by the Leukemia Society of America. Runners sign up to participate in one of the many marathons that Team in Training sends people to. In exchange for raising a specified amount of money (usually in the neighborhood of $3,000) in pledges, program participants receive free entry, travel, and lodging at their chosen marathon. The locales can be pretty exotic, such as the program's most popular race, the Mayor's Midnight Sun Marathon in Anchorage, Alaska. Other big Team in Training sites are Bermuda, Honolulu, San Diego, Dublin, and Paris.

Footnotes

Team in Training has had an incredible impact on the size of the field in some marathons. In 1994, just more than 300 people ran the Mayor's Midnight Sun Marathon in Anchorage, Alaska. In 1997, nearly 3,000 people ran the race, almost all of them Team in Training runners.

Runners in the program receive free coaching from knowledgeable runners in their area. Most groups meet once a week for a long run and a pre-run clinic from their coach. The usual training program lasts for six months so that the runners gradually build up to being able to finish the marathon.

Rules of the Road
Although some people run a marathon just six months after starting to run, I think you should wait until you've been running regularly for at least a year until you attempt this most demanding of distances. Give yourself a chance to build a solid base of endurance, and you'll be better able to increase your training toward a marathon.

Team in Training has been phenomenally successful in meeting its goals; it has raised more than $25 million for leukemia research, and now is the source of more than half of the Leukemia Society's revenue. Similar groups have sprung up that raise money for arthritis research (Joints in Motion) and cancer research (Fred's Team).

Many runners join these groups for emotional reasons—they know someone who suffers from the disease that their fundraising will battle. Almost all of the participants in these programs are first-time marathoners. In some cases, they're even first-time runners, having started to run only after deciding to finish a marathon to raise money for charity.

Charity runners care mostly about finishing their marathon to raise money, not how fast they can run the marathon. They've added an important new element to the sport and have helped running to continue to grow. (About 14,000 people take part in Team in Training each year.) Because of the good coaching they receive, nearly all of them complete their marathon. For more information, contact the groups directly: Team in Training, (800) 482-8326; Joints in Motion, (404) 872-7100; Fred's Team, (212) 639-3326.

Mastering the Possibilities

Now that I'm past the age of 50, I can no longer run a 5K at the same pace that I used to be able to maintain in a marathon. But that doesn't depress me. Why? Because like a lot of runners, I've been reborn since I became a *masters runner*.

No matter how long you've been running, once you're 40 or older, you'll be called a masters runner. For long-time runners like me, the phrase makes a certain amount of sense—after all those years of putting in the miles, you've mastered how to keep at it and with enough interest that you're still showing up at races.

What's so great about masters running? There must be something to it because I know I'm not alone in finding my running revitalized by the turning of the clock. Competition for the top prizes in the masters category are among the toughest in running. Masters running has become such a big deal that the Indianapolis Life Insurance Company sponsors a circuit of races around the country that's open only to masters runners.

Track Talk
A *masters runner* is a runner age 40 or older.

Masters racing recognizes that no matter how intelligently you go about your running, it's a lot tougher to run fast when you're 45 than when you're 25. That's especially so for people who have been at it for a long time. Most runners reach their best performances in the first 8 to 12 years of running, regardless of the age at which they start. So if you start at a young age, by the time you're 40, your times in races are almost assured to be slower than they were in your early 30s.

This inevitable slowing with age can be pretty depressing if you don't have a way to deal with it. Say there were no age-group awards in races, but just prizes for the top 10. Who would ever have a chance to take home a trophy except for the young and the breathless? Even if you were never an award winner in your youth, how would you go about setting goals when you know that no matter how hard you work, you're never going to run as fast as you once could?

Enter masters running. With awards given out in five-year brackets, you're not forced to fight it out with the young bucks if taking home loot is part of the appeal of racing to you. Instead, it's just you and your contemporaries, who are more likely to have the body and schedule that you do than some just-out-of-college hotshot is. The age-group categories level the playing field.

More importantly, masters running does a tremendous job of keeping runners motivated enough to keep attending races by giving you a way to set goals. In the last few years of my 30s, I was a little bit adrift. I was no longer fast enough to duke it out with the top guys in most races, and I wasn't running as fast I used to, even though I was training as hard. It was tough to know how to assess my performances and how to set goals for future ones.

Training Tip
Many big races have clinics or expos the day before. These clinics often feature expert speakers on running, so they're worth attending if you want to learn more about running.

Rules of the Road
For races of 10 miles and longer, you should run at least two-thirds of the distance at least once in the three weeks before the race. For example, before a half-marathon (13.1 miles), you should run at least 9 miles at least once in the preceding three weeks.

But when I turned 40, suddenly there were all these masters records to aim for—I got to see how close I could get to what other runners past the age of 40 had done. Mentally, I wiped the slate clean. I concentrated on setting masters personal records and took each personal record as a new standard, rather than comparing it to my faster times from my 20s and 30s. I start fresh every time I enter a new five-year age group.

That kind of attitude helps to explain why in some races, more than half the runners are past the age of 40. They've figured out that they can continue to find meaning in their race performances by comparing them to what they have achieved recently. Racing gives them a fresh outlook and new goals to shoot for every few years. When you do that, you've found the fountain of youth, regardless of how old your birth certificate says you are.

The Least You Need to Know

➤ Going to races adds excitement and variety to your running.

➤ The challenge of racing for time provides focus and motivation for your running.

➤ An increasing number of runners in marathons participate more to raise money for charity than to get a good finishing time.

➤ Comparing results within five-year age groups helps to keep a lot of runners coming back to races.

The Racing Circuit

In This Chapter

➤ The different types of races

➤ The cost of entering road races

➤ Finding races in your area

Arriving at a race can be an eerie experience. You may have been driving through early morning darkness for an hour, following directions from a photocopied race flyer that have taken you places you've never been before. When you get to the end of the directions, you start looking around, and you see them: Emerging from their cars, other runners are walking purposefully into that old school or that tent across the field. They've all somehow found their way from their homes to this one spot, where all of you will work together to get the best from yourselves. In this chapter, I'll show you how to join the party.

A Race to the Start: Types of Races

The different types of races are defined mainly by the type of surface they're run on. (Within each type are races of various distances.) You either race on the roads, on the track, or on dirt and grass. You rarely see a race that combines surfaces. Each of the different types of races has a feel all its own.

Takin' It to the Streets

More than 90 percent of the non-scholastic races held in the United States are road races. If you know someone who has run a race, it's almost guaranteed that he or she ran in a road race. There are road races of pretty much every distance you can imagine from the mile to the marathon. The most popular distances are 5K (3.1 miles), 8K (about 50 yards short of 5 miles), and 10K (6.2 miles).

The size of the fields in road races runs the gamut, too: You can find small rural affairs among 15 people all the way up to the country's biggest road race in terms of official entrants, The Lilac Bloomsday Run, a 12K (7.4 miles) run by more than 55,000 every May in Spokane, Washington. (Bay to Breakers, a 12K held every May in San Francisco, sometimes has as many as 100,000 people running it, but only about half of them have registered for the race.) A typical road race, in which runners wear race numbers and receive T-shirts, will have anywhere from a few hundred to 1,000 runners in it. Races with more than 1,000 runners are major productions.

I'm obviously biased toward road races, having earned the nickname "King of the Roads" in the '70s. I like how the course of each road race has its own quirks that you have to master. I also like the (usually) firm footing and long stretches so that I can get in a good rhythm. The party atmosphere that I told you so many races have is almost exclusively at road races.

Another cool aspect of road races is that they are one of the few, if not the only, instances in sports where an average participant competes at the same time on the same course as the best in the world. Want to play baseball with Cal Ripken? Good luck. But line up with the 50,000 runners who run the Peachtree 10K in Atlanta every Fourth of July, and some of the fastest runners around are at the front of the field. Sure, you're not going to be going head to head with them, but running is different because you're experiencing the race exactly as the elite runners do. It's fun to see how your time compares to theirs. You can't do that in baseball, football, basketball, or almost any other sport.

Choose Your Road

For the most part, road races basically fall into two main categories: those put on by various community organizations and those put on by local running clubs. The most popular time for both types of road races to be held is early on a weekend morning. Start time is usually 9 a.m. in the cooler months, 8 a.m. in the warmer months. More races are held on Sundays than on Saturdays.

Races in the first category are usually held in conjunction with a local event or as a once-a-year fundraiser for a charity. The people involved in organizing the race are usually volunteers from whatever organization will benefit from the race. The organizers usually pay a professional finish-line coordinator to handle timing, scoring, and other race-day logistics. In these races, you almost always wear a number during the race, and you almost always get a T-shirt as part of your entry fee. There's probably also going to be nice post-race refreshments, decent prizes for the top runners, and other amenities.

Local running clubs also put on races as part of their regular schedule of events. These races are usually more low-key and have smaller fields. Most of the people running them are members of the club, although all runners are certainly welcome to take part. Organization and logistics are handled entirely by volunteers lined up from the club. These races often cost only a few dollars to enter, because there are no T-shirts or other major costs to cover. (These races often take place in more rural areas, so the organizers don't have to pay as much, if anything, for permits, police, and so on.)

Training Tip

Many large races offer a way to pick up your race number on the day before the race. If doing so isn't a major hassle for you, this is a good way to avoid long lines on race day. Avoiding the long lines gives you the time and mental energy to focus on your race.

Footnotes

Does this race count as a morning or evening race? Every year at midnight on New Year's Eve, more than 5,000 runners take part in a 5K in New York City's Central Park.

Show Me the Money

Ted Poulos, of McLean, Virginia, runs more than 200 races a year. When you figure that the average race costs between $15 and $25 to enter, Ted has found himself an expensive little habit. Why do road races cost that much? I mean, aren't you just running down a public road? Who's getting rich off of these things?

Nobody is. The entry fee that races charge usually covers only about one third of the costs of putting on races. Events are a lot more expensive to stage than they used to be. Local governments didn't use to charge for the police who are often necessary for traffic control. Municipalities are also increasingly requiring races to pay for permits to stage events, even though there's really not a whole lot of demand for the space by others at 8 a.m. on Sundays. San Francisco's Bay to Breakers race shells out $30,000 for police services, plus $50,000 for park fees.

Rules of the Road

Races don't just get put on by magic. Any runner who attends races should volunteer at a race at least once a year. Volunteering at races is a good way for injured runners to stay connected to their sport.

Track Talk
Bandits are runners who participate in races without paying to register for them. Bandits like to think that they're protesting the high cost of races, but they're really cheapskates who hurt their fellow runners.

Training Tip
Registering early for a race is a good way to make a commitment to doing the race. Don't wait until you wake up on race day to decide whether you feel like going to the race. You almost never will.

Track Talk
A track meet that encourages runners of all speeds and ages to participate is an *all comer's meet.*

Most of the expenses to put on a race are picked up by the race sponsors. Donations also go a long way to keeping race costs down. Because most races are to benefit some charity or nonprofit group, the organizers can appeal to the good-will of local merchants to donate food and prizes. Given all that goes into putting on a race, a $20 entry fee is quite a bargain.

Some runners try to rebel against what they think are high entry fees by being *bandits*. They run the race, but don't sign up for it. Bandits are bad. Not only do they sometimes mess up the timing of the race because they're not wearing numbers, but they leech off of the majority of the runners who paid the entry fee. If everyone acted that way, then there wouldn't be any races for them to be mad at. If you think that a race charges too much, then voice your disagreement with a letter and by staying away, not by being a bandit and thinking that you're accomplishing anything more than ripping off fellow runners.

You can usually save money on races by registering a month or more before the race. Race day entry fees are usually about $5 higher than early registration.

Get on Track

Races held on the track can be hard to find once you're out of school. But especially during the summer, many local running clubs will put on one or more *all comer's meets.* In some parts of the country, you also can find indoor track meets open to all runners during the winter. These track meets are usually sparsely populated events, with less than 100 runners taking part. There are no T-shirts, and the entry fee is nominal. All comer's meets have an intimate atmosphere that's hard to match at a big road race.

Whereas road races are often about doing the best you can on the course you find yourself on, there's no such mystery in track races. Seen one, you've seen them all. Because of this universality of tracks, most runners are going to be there to chase after a time goal. As a result, many runners are intimidated by track races because they associate racing on the track with something that only really fast people do. That's a shame, because I think all racers should experiment with different types of races occasionally.

Track races are usually shorter than road races; 5K (12.5 laps of the track) is usually the longest race. Many runners gravitate to the longer distances because that's what's available on the road. But by running track races in addition to road races, you might find that you have a talent for speed-based events such as the mile.

Track races are also a good place to develop a strong sense of pace. Because there's no variation from lap to lap, you do best by getting in a rhythm. Learning how to get in a rhythm can help you on flat road courses as well. You also develop the ability to concentrate when you compete on the track frequently because churning lap after lap can get so boring.

Over Hill, Over Dale

The most elemental of races is *cross-country*. These races take place on grass and dirt, usually through woods, on golf courses, or in other pleasant settings. Cross-country races are usually from 5K to 10K in length and are usually held in the fall. Like track races, they're usually put on by local running clubs and have, at most, a couple of hundred runners. They usually are low-key affairs with no T-shirts and a small entry fee. Cross-country races are often team races, and many people like that aspect of them.

Times are pretty meaningless in cross-country, so runners concentrate on feeling that they ran strongly. Building on this attitude is the growing number of trail races. These races are usually much longer than standard cross-country races; sometimes they're as long as 50 miles or more. In spirit, these races are more akin to marathons, as most of the participants care more about finishing honorably than getting a certain time.

Track Talk
A race that's held on dirt or grass is a *cross-country* race.

Training for and racing cross-country can do a lot to help you as a runner on other surfaces. You learn to run strongly over uneven terrain, and you become a better hill runner. Kenyan men have won the team title at the World Cross-Country Championships every year since 1986, and every year they produce an astonishing percentage of the top track and road runners in the world.

Footnotes

My first race at a world-class level was a cross-country race. In March 1975, I placed third in the World Cross-Country Championships. A month later, I supposedly "came out of nowhere" to win the Boston Marathon for the first time, but one of the reasons I knew I was ready to run a good marathon was because of my good cross-country race.

How to Find a Race

Where can you find details on races in your area? The best place to start is with a local running club. Don't worry if you don't know anyone in the club or even how to contact them. If you don't know any runners in your area who you can ask about local clubs, call the national office of the Road Runners Club of America at (703) 836-0558. Ask for the name and number of the club nearest to you. Once you know the club in your area, give it a call. Most clubs maintain a hotline that has a recording of upcoming club races.

Training Tip
Arrive at the site of a race 45 minutes to an hour before the start. This will give you time to park, register, find a bathroom, and warm up with plenty of time to spare and without worrying that you're going to miss the start.

If you know of a running store near you, visit it. Ask the salespeople (who are usually local runners) if they know where you can find information about local races. Many areas have local running publications that do a fantastic job of listing all of the upcoming races in a locale. Most running stores are also depositories for race flyers. Look through them to see if any of them interest you.

If you have Internet access, next stop is the World Wide Web. Appendix B, "Resources for Runners," lists some of the best running Web sites. Because of the nature of this book, most of those Web sites are national in scope, but many have links to local running Web sites. There, you can often find race listings.

The two top national running magazines, *Runner's World* and *Running Times*, list upcoming races in their calendar sections. Of the two, *Running Times* maintains a more in-depth calendar, but neither can possibly list all of the 15,000 races that are held in the United States every year. Their calendars are handy resources, however, if you're going to be traveling and want to sneak in a race while you're away.

Seasons in the Sun

The best runners in the world take a seasonal approach to their racing year. For example, they'll focus on cross-country races in the winter, road races in the spring, and then shorter track races in the summer. In the fall, they might run more road races or take a break from racing. Top marathoners aim for one or two peak marathons a year, using shorter races at other times of the year as part of their buildup to their next marathon. When I raced marathons, I usually made a spring marathon, such as the Boston Marathon in April, one focus. When I recovered from that, I'd run shorter races as I built back up to a fall marathon, such as the New York City Marathon.

Many recreational runners could benefit from this approach, but the current racing calendar can make it tough. It's so darned enticing! As running has become more popular, races have proliferated like *Star Trek* TV series—it seems that no matter where you look, you see one. Still, in parts of the country that have definite seasons, at least a bit of logic remains in what races are offered when. After all, a marathon is tough enough by itself. You don't need a hot summer day to add your work.

Here's when some of the most popular races are most often held:

Rules of the Road

If it's 80 degrees or warmer at the start of a race, start the race slower than you had planned. The heat is going to take its toll on you regardless, so it's better that you be in control of the situation rather than overheating and slowing down even more.

➤ Although 5K road races are held pretty much year round, you might do better in them in warmer months, because it can be tough to get going quickly when it's cold.

➤ Although 8K to 10K road races are also held year round, their popularity peaks in spring and fall because even 10K can get too long in hot weather.

➤ Because runners build toward marathons and concentrate on longer runs in the cooler months, 10-milers and half-marathons are mostly held in the fall and winter.

➤ Marathons are mostly held in the fall, with the spring being the second most popular time. Summer is out of the question in many places.

As I mentioned earlier, most track meets are held in the summer, and cross-country races are usually held in the fall.

The Least You Need to Know

➤ The three main types of races are road races, track meets, and cross-country races.

➤ Road races are by far the most popular type of race.

➤ The average road race is between 5K and 10K long, costs $15 to $25 to enter, and is held early on a weekend morning.

➤ The best sources for information on races in your area are local running clubs and running stores.

Basic Training for Racers

In This Chapter

➤ Reasons to vary the length and pace of your runs

➤ Tips on how to schedule different runs within a week

➤ Advice on how to run fast and relaxed at the same time

➤ Guidelines for speed-building workouts

Getting out the door for 30 or so minutes of steady running a few times a week brings you most of the health benefits. But if you want to run faster in races, you need to add some extra elements to your training. In this chapter, I'll show the types of workouts that I and other racers do to improve our performance, and I'll show you how to fit them all together into a sensible plan.

I'm going to be throwing a lot of lingo at you in this chapter. Just like on a hard run, don't feel bad if you need to slow down and catch your breath. At the end of this chapter, even if you never do any of these workouts, you'll at least be able to hold up your end of the conversation with any running geek.

Adding More Structure

Nobody needs to do the workouts in this chapter. You can run the same distance at the same pace every day for the rest of your life, and I'll gladly call you a fellow runner. Certainly no one has ever been barred from entering a race because they hadn't done hard workouts on the track for the last several weeks.

But if you want to run faster in races and your running is at the moderate, steady pace that I've been urging, you need to make a few changes in your training. You'll race better if once a week you include a few miles of running at race pace or faster. You'll have more strength for these fast workouts if you boost your endurance by occasionally running longer than usual.

A lot of runners avoid doing this type of training because they don't like the idea of planning their running so meticulously. They just want to get out the door and run how they feel on a given day. They think that adding more structure to their running will make it less interesting.

Training Tip
When you add more structure, plot your training a week at a time so that you're sure to allow enough time between your hardest efforts. Be realistic about when you'll have the time and energy to do which workouts. A common plan is to do your longest run of the week on Saturday or Sunday and your fastest workout in the middle of the week.

Actually, the opposite is true. Variety is the spice of running as well as life. When you add different types of workouts to your running, then you've gone a long way toward finding a way to keep yourself motivated from day to day. Each run seems to have more of a purpose. If I've done a fast workout on the track on a Wednesday, then I look forward to running slowly on the roads on Thursday to recover. By the weekend, I'm looking forward to joining some friends for my longest run on the week, which I'll look forward to following the next day with a short, slow run by myself, which will get me fired up for that track workout on Wednesday, and so on.

I think all runners, even those who aren't going to race, should at least dabble in the different types of workouts covered in this chapter. Including runs that are faster or longer than usual is just part of training more completely, like stretching and strengthening exercises are.

The Hard-Easy Principle

In Chapter 3, I told you that you progress in your running by applying a stress, allowing enough recovery time for your body to rebuild itself a little stronger, and then applying a slightly higher stress. When you start adding different types of workouts, apply that principle to your training as a whole. You want to start training by the hard-easy principle—you run faster or longer than usual on one day, and then follow that day with a run that's shorter or slower than usual.

The hard-easy principle helps you in two connected ways. Say I have a fast track workout planned for Wednesday. On Tuesday, I'll be sure to run very easy. This might mean running a bit less than usual, and it definitely means running at a slow pace for the entire run, no matter how good I feel. This slow pace reserves my body's strength for the next day and allows me to have a better workout than if I had gone into it more tired. By running easy before a hard effort, you progress because you're able to get more out of yourself on your hard days.

For at least one day after my fast workout on Wednesday, and more often two days, I'll take it easy again. After a hard workout, it's usually easy to go slow enough because I'm beat from the previous day's work. Taking it easy allows me to consolidate the gains from my hard workout and helps me to avoid injury. If you run too fast or long on the day after a hard workout, then you're risking injury or staleness later on. Your body needs that chance to rebuild itself.

Remember that the general rule is to plan an easy day the day before a hard workout and allow for at least one or two easy days after a hard workout. By hard workout I mean either a run that includes at least a couple of miles at race pace or faster or a run that's much longer than usual. What counts as an easy day varies among runners. For some runners, an easy day means a day of no running—that's certainly a good way to make sure you don't work too hard! In running terms, an easy day means making sure that you can pass the talk test the entire run.

Before and after fast running, it's OK to run your usual distance, as long as you keep the pace easy. Before and after runs that are longer than usual, you should not only keep the pace easy, but also run a shorter distance than usual. The longer runs drain your glycogen stores. The day before, you don't want to run too far because you might start your long run low on glycogen. The day after a long run, your muscles will still be a little low on fuel, so you're risking injury if you ask them to go too far.

Track Talk
Striders are runs of 100 yards or so done at close to top speed. Striders help you learn how to stay relaxed when you run fast.

Smooth Striding

One of the best ways to introduce fast running into your program is by doing *striders*. Striders are good because they're fast enough to teach your muscles and nervous system how to run smoothly at a fast pace, but they're so short that they don't fatigue you.

Striders don't really count as a hard workout. Still, I think that all runners should do them once or twice a week. Striders move you through a fuller range of motion than regular moderate runs. They also feel great—it's fun to run at close to top speed, knowing that you're only going to be doing so for 20 seconds or so.

Most runners do striders at or near the end of a normal run. When you do striders, do 8 to 12. Some runners like to do them on the straightaway of a track, so they know that they're going about 100 yards and that the footing will be good. But you can do them anywhere you can run smoothly for 100 yards at a time on a flat, level surface. A good day to do striders is the day before a fast workout or a long run. Striders wake up your body from the usual plodding. That's why most serious runners also do a few striders just before starting a fast workout or a race.

The key to doing striders is to stay relaxed. Watch the top sprinters in the world, and you'll see that although they're running faster than 25 miles per hour, their entire bodies, especially their shoulders, neck, and face, are incredibly relaxed. Shoot for this lack of tension when you do striders. Accelerate smoothly to what feels like the fastest pace you could maintain for half a mile. Try to reach that speed by halfway, hold that speed for a bit, and then gradually slow down. Wait a minute or so, and then start your next strider.

Striders are a great way to improve your running form. By learning to run smoothly when you're running at close to top speed, you become better able to do so at all speeds. On each strider, concentrate on one aspect of good running form. For example, concentrate on keeping your shoulders low and relaxed during one strider. On the next, think about maintaining a quick, smooth turnover of your feet. On the next, concentrate on keeping your hands cupped, relaxed, and passing your body at about your waist. Pretty soon, you've done your 8 to 12 striders.

The Long and Short of Long Runs

When I was training to be the best marathoner in the world, my *long run* was the focus of my week. But you don't have to be a marathoner to benefit from long runs, and your long runs don't have to be 20 miles or more, like mine were. What counts as a long run is relative to how much you usually run. Marathoners need to build up to at least a couple of runs of 20 miles or more before they should try to cover 26.2 miles. But for a 5K runner, a long run could be as short as six miles.

Track Talk
A *long run* is a run that's at least one and a half times longer than your second longest run of the week. For a runner who usually runs five miles at a time, eight miles is a long run. Most runners do a long run every one to two weeks.

There's no set standard for what constitutes a long run, but here's a good guideline: Two out of every three weeks, do a run that's at least one and a half times longer than any other run you do that week. If your normal run is three miles, then five miles is a long run for you. Hard-core runners who log 10 miles a day would say that they're "going long" if they went 15 miles or more. If you measure your runs by time, the same standard applies. If you usually run for half an hour, then going 45 minutes or more would be a long run for you.

Many runners do a long run every week, but you don't have to. Two out of every three weeks is a good goal. This frequency is enough to progress in boosting your endurance, but the occasional week off gives you a chance to recoup physically and mentally. A plan that many runners use is to do a long run on weekends that they're not racing. This plan mixes things up nicely.

What do you get from doing long runs? Obviously, marathoners need to train their bodies and minds to be out there for a long time. But every runner, even ones who aren't going to race, should incorporate runs of varying lengths into their training. When you do a long run, you deplete your muscles' glycogen stores more than usual. During your recovery from the long run, your muscles develop the ability to store more glycogen. This means that the next time you run as far, your muscles won't get tired as soon.

Footnotes

Other things happen in your muscle cells when you do long runs that help you on all of your runs. Capillaries, the tiniest blood vessels, border every muscle fiber. Their job is to deliver oxygen and fuel to your muscles and take away waste products. Long runs increase the number of capillaries per muscle fiber, which improves their efficiency. This increased efficiency makes all of your runs feel easier. Also, long runs increase the number and size of mitochondria in your muscle cells. (Mitochondria are the little aerobic energy factories in your muscles.) With more mitochondria, you can produce more energy, so you can maintain a faster pace at a given level of effort.

Psychologically, long runs help your usual runs seem easier. When you're used to being out there for almost an hour once a week, then your normal 30-minute runs don't seem as daunting. And obviously, the longer you run, the more calories you burn, and the longer you'll burn calories at an accelerated rate after your run. Long runs are great for losing weight.

Do your long runs at your normal training pace. These runs count as hard workouts because of the increased distance, not because you maintain a faster pace. You should be able to finish your long runs at the same pace you start them. If you have to slow dramatically at the end, then you've prematurely depleted your glycogen stores by starting too quickly.

Rules of the Road

If you've been nursing a slight injury but are still going to try a long run, create a course that keeps you close to home, such as several different small loops. That way, if your injury flares up, you can cut your run short more easily.

The key to successfully increasing your long run is progressing gradually. When you can comfortably complete a long run at a given distance, try going one mile farther the next time. This is the approach I take. After my racing season ends in the fall, I take it easy for a while. My longest run for a month will be 10 miles or so. Starting in December, I'll go 12 miles or so once a week, and then start adding one mile per long run until I'm at my target distance.

Make your long runs special. Try to do them in a nice setting, and try to do them with friends. These factors will make these runs more enjoyable, and the miles will pass more easily.

Warming Up and Cooling Down

You should start all of your runs at a gentle pace and spend the first 5 to 10 minutes of the run building to your normal training pace. This gradual building allows your muscles, heart, and lungs to warm up and work better when you want to get going. You also should ease off during the last bit of a run to allow your heart rate to return to normal more gradually. When you start doing races and fast workouts like the ones in this chapter, you need to make your warm-up and *cool-down* much more pronounced.

Track Talk
A *cool-down* is running very easily for one to three miles after a fast workout or race. A cool-down helps to remove some of the waste products that build in your muscles when you run hard, so cool-downs help you to recover from a hard run more quickly.

Most people know that they should warm up before trying to do something hard, whether it's running fast, lifting a heavy weight, or what have you. The best way to warm up for any activity is by doing that activity at a low level of effort. So a weightlifter might do a few bench presses at a very low weight, and runners might run one to three miles very slowly before they try to run fast.

Where many runners fall short is on the other end of the workout. They neglect to do a good cool-down after a hard effort. Usually that's because they're exhausted, and think that more running is just going to exhaust them more.

But cooling down (you'll also hear runners call it warming down, but that's really the opposite of what you're doing) helps you recover more quickly from your hard efforts. When you finish a race or a hard workout, your heart rate is near its maximum, and waste products have built up in your muscles. You're tired, so you plop down and consider yourself done for the day. The next time you run, your legs are still sore because those waste products have pooled in your muscles. A good cool-down flushes those waste products out.

Cool-downs don't have to be long. One mile is often plenty. After catching your breath, run very slowly for at least 10 minutes. A cool-down run should be at a much slower pace than your regular runs. By the end of the cool-down, I guarantee that you'll feel better.

On the Fast Track: Speed Work

Speed work is the best way to train the physiological systems that are stressed when you race. Your regular daily runs give you the base to cover the distance; striders help you to run fast smoothly; long runs give you a little extra boost of endurance so that you can keep running strong when you get tired. But to boost your performance in a race, you need to do some running at the pace that you hope to maintain in the race or even a little bit faster.

Track Talk
Speed work is running a workout of several runs of a mile or shorter at race pace or faster, with slow recovery jogs between the hard runs.

Running fast works in the same general way as running long does. After you do a long run, your body rebuilds itself so that it's better prepared the next time that you try to do such a silly thing. Same thing with running fast—your leg muscles get more used to turning over quickly, your heart gets used to working at a higher rate for a sustained time, and your lungs get used to processing a lot more oxygen. Just as important, your mind gets used to putting up with a certain kind of pain, but persisting nonetheless.

When you do speed work at the right intensity, you're going to be near your maximum effort. A little voice (OK, sometimes it's huge) inside your head will beg you to get off this crazy ride. You'll learn how to keep this voice at bay as you become more used to pushing yourself to keep running fast despite your fatigue. By combining the physical and mental benefits of speed work, you'll be able to sustain a faster pace in your races.

Aim for one speed workout a week when you're building toward a race. The best ways to make speed work more bearable are to stay focused on your race goal to remind yourself why you're doing it and (does this sound familiar?) to do speed work with others of similar ability (see the following figure). Many runners who run on their own every other day of the week seek out people to do speed workouts with. They know that they'll be less likely to bag the workout when they're running with others, and they know that sharing the effort with others helps the workout to pass more quickly.

Footnotes

Top runners have long known the value of doing their fastest workouts with others. Kyle Heffner made the Olympic Marathon team in 1980. While training for that race, Heffner drove three hours round-trip once a week just to have company on his speed work.

Speed workouts are easier when you do them with other runners.

A Decent Interval

Track Talk

Intervals are structured speed work in which you run fast for a specified distance, run very slowly for a specified time or distance to recover, and then repeat the process a specified number of times. Different interval workouts are best to prepare for different races.

The most popular place to do speed work is at a standard 400-meter outdoor track. Such a track is precise and unvarying, so you get objective feedback about how fast you're running. When you do speed work on the track, you're doing *intervals*.

An interval workout has a defined structure. First, you run fast for a specified distance (usually one to four laps, which equals one-quarter to one mile). You have a rest interval of a set length, expressed either in distance or time, during which you jog very easily to recover from the fast run. At the end of that interval, you run fast again. You repeat this process for the number of times you had planned at the start of your workout.

Technically, the term *intervals* refer to the recovery portion of the workout, but everyone has his or her own usage for this term. Some people call the fast runs the intervals, as in, "I'm going to do mile intervals today." (I will use the term this way in this book.) Other people don't use the intervals term at all; they call the fast runs repeats, as in, "I'm going to do half-mile repeats today." Don't let them confuse you. If they talk about doing intervals, that refers to the workout as a whole; it means they're doing speed work on the track. (Some runners just say they're "doing a workout," meaning that they're going to do intervals as opposed to a normal training run.)

Most runners do intervals of one to four laps. As Chapter 4 explained, doing intervals that are one lap long is called doing quarters, because a 400-meter track is just short of a quarter-mile long. That's a standard distance for intervals, but for the wrong reason. It seems so logical to do one lap fast at a time, so quarters have become a regular part of many people's training. But unless you're going to be racing the mile, quarters don't help most runners as much as longer intervals do.

Quarters are too short to require any real sustained effort, so you have to do tons of them to get the benefits that you get from fewer numbers of longer intervals. When you do longer intervals, such as two laps or four laps, you're working at the intensity that's going to be required of you in races for a longer period of time on each interval. Running fast for a longer time provides a better stress to your system.

How do you structure an interval workout? What's best depends on what race you're training for. If you're concentrating on 5Ks, then you're better off running shorter intervals at a slightly higher intensity. If you're getting ready for a half-marathon, you should do longer intervals at a bit slower pace.

In the next three chapters, I'll show you what interval workouts are best for the most popular race distances. Here are some general guidelines:

> **Training Tip**
> If you're working out at a track with others, take turns leading. Have each member of the group lead an entire hard run. Switching the lead allows you to draft off of someone, so you don't have to work as hard to maintain the pace, and it breaks the workout up psychologically.

> **Rules of the Road**
> If other people are on the track during your speed workouts, do your recovery jogs in the outside lanes so that you don't get in their way.

➤ Aim for a total of 15 to 20 minutes of hard running in your workout. This range means that the shorter your intervals, the more you should do of them. Don't do more than 25 minutes total of hard running in a single workout.

➤ For intervals that take longer than five minutes to complete, allow a recovery time of about 50 percent of the time it took you to complete the interval. For example, if you run a fast mile in eight minutes, recover for four minutes before running hard again.

221

➤ For intervals that take from three to five minutes to complete, allow a recovery of about 75 percent of the time it took you to complete the interval. For example, if you run a fast half-mile in 3:30, recover for 2:30 before running hard again.

➤ For intervals that take less than three minutes to complete, allow a recovery time that lasts roughly as long as it took you to complete the interval. For example, if you run a fast quarter-mile in 1:40, recover for 1:40 before running hard again.

➤ Have the workout planned before you start. If you make it up as you go along, you're more likely to quit too early.

➤ Figure out what your goal pace for an interval is in terms of time per lap, and then try to hit that pace on each lap. For example, if you want to run each of your interval miles in eight minutes, try to run each lap as close to two minutes as possible.

➤ Your time from interval to interval shouldn't vary by more than 10 seconds per mile. If you run two interval miles in 8:00 each, and then a third one in 8:30, you did the first two too quickly.

Track Talk
Running a speed workout in which the fast parts vary in length is called running a *ladder*.

Training Tip
Bring water with you to the track on hot days. Taking a small drink between your hard efforts is a nice mental break and will help you feel better on your intervals.

How fast to run depends on how long your intervals are. I'll show you how to figure that pace for specific workouts in the next three chapters.

Some runners add variety to their interval workouts by doing a *ladder*, or varying the distance of the intervals. The name comes from the visual image of going up in distance, and then coming back down by the end of the workout. For example, you might run two quarters, and then a half-mile interval, and then a mile interval to finish the climb up the ladder. Then you would come back down as you went up, with a half-mile interval and two quarters.

Ladders can help to break up a workout psychologically. You can tell yourself, "OK, just one hard mile, and then they all get shorter the rest of the workout." If you sometimes need to coax yourself into finishing your speed work, ladders can be helpful. In general, though, it's better to stick with intervals of one distance so that you practice pushing yourself mentally as your fatigue increases. That's certainly how it happens in races!

Fartlek: Not an Intestinal Disorder

Some runners thrive on track workouts. They love the precision and the ability to objectively compare their workouts from week to week. A lot of runners get burned out when they do speed work on the track frequently, however. They just don't like going around and around in circles. Also, many runners don't have easy access to a track, or they have to train when it's dark, or the track is covered with snow. How can these runners get in their fast running?

They can do *fartlek*. That's not what you do on a run after having a burrito; it's a Swedish word that translates as "speed play." Fartlek workouts are done away from the track. Many runners prefer them because the change in scenery makes them less mentally grinding, and they find that they can concentrate of running fast.

Fartleks can be a lot less structured than speed work on the track. You might plan a fartlek on your usual five-mile course. After running easily for a mile, you might run hard to that telephone pole way down the street, and then jog easily until the end of the next block, and then pick up the pace again until the school, and so on until you had a mile left in your run, when you would run easy the rest of the way home as your cool-down.

Some runners make fartleks more structured. They might head out on one of their loops and, after warming up, spend the bulk of their run alternating running hard for two minutes with running easy for two minutes. Runners who don't have access to a track often use this approach. (It helps to have an alarm on your watch for this type of workout.) This approach is also good when the weather is bad, and you know it would be hard to reach your usual times on the track. In this situation, do a fartlek on the roads and get in a good workout without the weather-induced slower times bumming you out.

> **Track Talk**
> *Fartlek* is a Swedish word that means "speed play." When you do a fartlek workout, you alternate fast and slow running, but you do the workout on roads or trails rather than the track. Fartlek workouts are usually less structured than track workouts.

> **Footnotes**
> Steve Jones set a world record for the marathon in 1984 and almost never trained on the track. Nearly all of his fast running workouts were fartlek sessions on the road.

Doing fartleks on the road is a good choice if you're going to be running road races with hills in them. If you do all of your fast running on the track, then you might not be able to tackle the uphills in races as well. But if you're alternating running hard for three minutes with running slow for two minutes on a road course, then you'll go over more varied terrain. Sometimes, you might start running hard at the base of a hill. Or your recovery jog might end when you're halfway down a hill. You'll learn how to keep running strongly off of the flat.

Fartleks are a safer way to run fast on hills than what some runners do, which is a series of intervals of running fast up a hill, and then jogging down to recover. Sure, this workout is very effective, but it also increases your risk of injury. If you want to work on your hill running ability, do fartleks on the road, and do your long runs on hilly courses.

The Least You Need to Know

➤ You'll progress more in your running if you regularly vary the lengths and paces of your runs.

➤ A long run once a week builds your endurance and makes your regular runs easier.

➤ Alternating very fast running with slow recovery jogs is speed work.

➤ To race your best, you need to do speed work regularly.

➤ You can do speed work on a track, road, or trail.

Chapter 20

Short but Sweet: 5Ks to 10Ks

In This Chapter

➤ Maximizing your aerobic capacity

➤ Learn why you should run at an even pace in your races

➤ Training schedule for 5K races

➤ Training schedule for 8K/10K races

More people run 5K (3.1 miles) races than any other distance. The second most popular races are 10Ks (6.2 miles). In recent years, an intermediate distance has become increasingly popular—8K, or about 50 yards short of 5 miles.

What's so great about these races? You don't have to train like a marathoner to run them, and they're not going to leave you walking downstairs backward for days afterward, but they're still very challenging distances. You're running right at the limits of your aerobic capacity, seeing whether you can hang on for just a bit longer until the finish line comes into view.

If you want to know how to improve your performance at these distances, this chapter is for you. I'll show you how to set goals for these races and give you an eight-week schedule leading up to a target race.

How Far Is a K?

What's the deal with all these "K"s runners are always talking about? I mean, everyone trains all week by measuring their miles, and then they go off on the weekend and race 5Ks and 10Ks. "K" stands for kilometer, as in a five-kilometer race. A kilometer is a metric standard of distance equal to 1,000 meters. One kilometer equals .621 miles.

Europe is the epicenter of the international track and field circuit. Every summer, the best runners in the world spend June through August traveling to track meets throughout Europe to race each other. World-class track meets in Europe are like the Super Bowl is here. They often sell out more than a year in advance, with some stadiums holding more than 50,000 fans.

I ran a few of these meets in the late '70s, and it was an incredible experience. The fans are really knowledgeable. They spend most of the distance races clapping rhythmically, stomping their feet, cheering wildly. You can't help drawing from their energy. You just don't see that happening at track meets in this country, which are usually more sparsely attended than a shoe-sniffing contest.

Footnotes

When this book went to print, the men's and women's world records for 5K on the track were 12:39, by Daniel Komen of Kenya, and 14:28, by Jiang Bo of China. That's 4:04 per mile for Komen and 4:39 per mile for Jiang. The American records are 12:58, by Bob Kennedy, and 14:56, by Amy Rudolph.

As a result, European track meets set the agenda. Because tracks are measured metrically, being 400 meters around, almost all races are in metric distances. (The main exception is the mile, which fans all over the world love.) The two main distance races are 5,000 meters, or 5K, and 10,000 meters, or 10K. Usually when people talk about track races, they give the distance in meters; when they talk about the same race on the roads, they describe it in kilometers. So a 5,000 on the track is the same distance as a 5K on the roads. Wacky, eh?

Road races used to be all kinds of strange distances: 4.7 miles, 7.1 miles, 11.6 miles, whatever. People would lay out a good course, measure it, and that's how far the race was. But when the first running boom started in the '70s, the new breed of runner wanted more precision. Theses runners wanted to be able to compare their times from week to week to make sure that their 5K time this month was better than it had been last month. So the standard distance races from the track were transported to the roads. Next thing you knew, runners who failed algebra could instantaneously convert miles to kilometers and back again.

But what about 8Ks, which are never run on the track? Why don't those races lengthen their course by 47 yards and call themselves five-milers? Wouldn't it be a lot easier to know what your pace in them was that way? I don't know. Stop asking so many questions. Just run 'em.

Racing 101

The first step to running your best in any race is being able to cover the distance. I don't care how fast Carl Lewis can sprint; if 5K is a long run for him, he's not beating me (or many other people, for that matter) in that race. The longer a race is, the more being able to negotiate the distance becomes a limiting factor. That's why 5Ks to 10Ks are so popular. You don't have to run all that many miles each week to be able to finish the race.

But when you want to do more than just finish the race, then you need to alter your training. How? Here's a simple training principle that many runners ignore: Different races have different physiological demands; that is, they stress different systems of your body. It's impossible to effectively train all of the systems of your body in a short period (say, a few months). Therefore, to reach your potential, you should pick a race distance that you want to focus on for a racing season, and then train to meet the physiological demands of your target race.

In other words, you can't train to be a miler and a marathoner at the same time. The demands of the distances are so different that you have to choose, and then structure your training accordingly. If you want to be a miler, then do a lot of short, very fast speed workouts, and don't worry about how many miles you run each week. If you want to be a marathoner, don't worry about how fast you can run a quarter-mile; concentrate on increasing your endurance with long runs.

Footnotes

When this book went to print, the men's and women's world records for 10K on the track were 26:27, by Paul Tergat of Kenya, and 29:31, by Wang Junxia of China. That's 4:15 per mile for Tergat and 4:45 per mile for Wang. The American records are 27:20, by Mark Nenow, and 31:19, by Lynn Jennings.

This focused, seasonal approach is what the best runners in the world do, but many recreational runners are all over the place. They run a 5K one weekend, a half marathon the next, then another 5K, then a 10K. That's not to say that you can't or shouldn't race at a variety of distances. But within any period of a few months, you'll do better if you focus on a group of distances that have similar physiological demands. That way, you'll be able to train more effectively because you can concentrate on developing the type of fitness needed for your target races.

This principle underlies the workouts that I recommend in the next three chapters. After all, 5Ks and 10Ks place different demands on you than marathons do. Therefore, the workouts that you do to prepare for them should be different. Otherwise, you're wasting valuable training time.

VO₂ to the Max

The key to training to become faster at 5Ks, 8Ks, and 10Ks is to improve your aerobic capacity, or VO_2 max. That's because you run these races at very close to your aerobic capacity—an all-out 5K is run at about 95 percent of your VO_2 max, a 10K at about 92 percent. To run those races better, then, you need to max out your VO_2 max. The best way to do that is to do one workout each week in which you run intervals at a pace that's roughly at your VO_2 max.

But wait a minute. Didn't I tell you early on in this book that steady, comfortable running increases your VO_2 max and that it will increase by 20 to 30 percent within a year of running? Why would you need to do anything more to race a good 5K? Early on, you don't. You're getting fitter by leaps and bounds just by running easy. But after those initial gains, you have to work harder to keep improving. It's like learning a new computer program—you make the greatest improvements in the beginning, when you go from complete unfamiliarity to a basic working knowledge. It's only after more extensive experience that you learn all those little tricks of the program that allow you to make that small but significant leap from a basic user to the one in the office who every one asks for advice.

In the training schedules at the end of this chapter, I'll have you do one speed workout each week that will focus on boosting your VO_2 max by having you run your intervals at roughly that pace. In your case, I'm making them a bit faster, because I'm assuming you haven't done systematic speed work before, so you have more room for improvement than a long-time runner. It's important to run them as close as possible to that pace to get the greatest improvement.

In these workouts, harder isn't necessarily better. Most runners think that if they can run a workout of three interval miles in 8:00, then running them in 7:40 will be that much more of an effective workout. But it doesn't always work that way. In these workouts, the important thing is to work right at the limits of your VO_2 max. But that's not the same as your max.

Remember, you run 5Ks very close to your VO_2 max. But obviously you can run shorter races faster; you can maintain a quicker pace for 1 mile than you can for 3.1 miles. In races shorter than 5K, a bigger percentage of your energy is supplied anaerobically, independent of the oxygen that you

Training Tip
It's common to feel suddenly tired soon before you have a speed workout planned. That feeling is almost always just nerves and anxiety about the hard work in front of you. Just go through a good warm-up, remind yourself how the workout will help you to reach your goals, and start the first interval.

breathe in. So it's possible to run faster than your VO2 max for a short distance, stop running until you catch your breath, and then run anaerobically again.

Unfortunately, many ambitious runners do their speed workouts this way. They run each interval as hard as they can. When they do that, they're definitely training hard, but they're not training very effectively. By training faster than their VO2 max pace, their workouts are more anaerobic, so they're training their anaerobic systems. But then they go and race 5Ks, 8Ks, and 10Ks, which rely almost entirely on their aerobic systems. In their races, they'll often not perform up to their expectations. They'll think, "Gee, I ran three mile intervals the other night in 7:00 each, but I could only average 7:20s in the race." To make matters worse, they'll then often think that this means that should train that much harder, and the next week they'll push themselves to run their mile intervals in 6:50.

See how they're making their workouts less and less effective the farther that they stray from doing them at their VO2 max pace? Don't let it happen to you. Train at the right intensity, and you can pass them in the races, leaving them to wonder why you're behind them in speed workouts, but ahead of them in races.

The Proper Pace Prescription

I've convinced you that you'll run faster in 5Ks to 10Ks by doing a weekly speed workout at your VO2 max pace, and I've convinced you that you'll improve more if you do them at this pace instead of as fast as you possibly can. Now you have just one question: How do you know what that pace is?

If you've run a 5K race at a solid effort within the last few months and have been running consistently since, use that pace as your current VO2 max pace. Better yet, hop in a 5K race soon, run hard the entire way, and figure out your average pace per mile. In both cases, make your 5K goal pace (what, you hope, will become your new VO2 max pace) about 15 seconds per mile faster. If you haven't run a 5K in a while (or ever), you can still figure out the proper pace. If you're running at least 15 miles per week and know your average training pace, subtract one minute per mile to get a reasonable 5K goal pace.

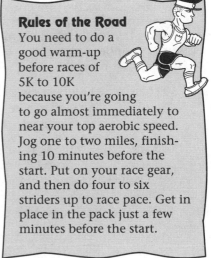

Rules of the Road
You need to do a good warm-up before races of 5K to 10K because you're going to go almost immediately to near your top aerobic speed. Jog one to two miles, finishing 10 minutes before the start. Put on your race gear, and then do four to six striders up to race pace. Get in place in the pack just a few minutes before the start.

The 5K and 10K training schedules later in this chapter include speed workouts that are based on your 5K goal pace. The intervals in the 8K/10K schedule are a little longer and a little slower to better meet the demands of the longer races. If you're decently trained, you should be able to run an 8K or 10K within 10 to 15 seconds per mile of your 5K race pace.

229

Track Talk
When you run so fast that you can't take in enough oxygen to meet your muscles' needs, you've gone into *oxygen debt*. When this happens, you either have to slow down or stop running. You can avoid going into oxygen debt by having the right goal pace, and then running that pace from the start of the race.

Track Talk
Running the second half of a race faster than the first half is called running *negative splits*.

These workouts will help you to know what pace to try to reach in your race. You'll be used to running hard while tired. After awhile, the pace will become second nature. That's not to say that it will feel easy, but that you can launch into it and be confident that you're at your goal pace until you get your first split time.

You should try to run as even a pace as you can in races of 5K to 10K. Many runners like to blast through the first mile much faster than their goal pace. This is a bad idea. Their reason behind doing this is to build a cushion to allow for when they slow later in the race, and their strategy becomes self-fulfilling. They have to slow in the second half of the race because they've gone into *oxygen debt*. Oxygen debt doesn't demonstrate how mentally tough they are; it is an unforgiving physiological fact of life. As a result, their overall time is slower than if they had run at an even pace.

In races of 5K to 10K, when you're working right at your VO_2 max, you have a very small margin of error. If you run more than 10 seconds per mile faster than your VO_2 max pace, then you're running at a pace that you can sustain for at most two miles, usually much less. Trouble is, you still have at least a mile to go. So you're going to have to slow way down, and you're really going to hurt. It's not uncommon for runners to have to slow by more than 30 seconds per mile in the last mile of a 5K when they've started too quickly.

In these short races, I sometimes start out a little bit more slowly than my goal pace. I give myself the first few minutes of the race to build gradually. For the first few minutes, I might be running at 5 to 10 seconds per mile slower than my goal pace. This slower start helps my heart and muscles better adapt to the sudden shock of running so quickly.

Then, when all systems are firing, I can take off. Running an even pace is physically the most efficient way to race, but trying to run *negative splits* provides a tremendous psychological boost. You're passing other runners pretty much the whole way.

If you've ever run a race and been passed by someone in the last mile, you know how disconcerting it can be. You're trying as hard as you can, and this runner is just blowing by you. There's nothing you can do. When I run negative splits, I like to key on a runner about 100 yards ahead of me. I'll focus on chasing him down and pulling him in gradually, and then I pass him quickly to demoralize him and move on to my next target.

Running at an even pace or at negative splits leaves you better prepared for your *kick*. How good a kick you'll have at the end of a 5K, 8K, or 10K depends a lot on how intelligently you ran the race. If you haven't gone out too quickly, then you'll still be running aerobically. This means that you can start your kick from farther out than if you've gone into oxygen debt. If you have good natural speed, you can shave several seconds from your finishing time with a good, long kick.

Your body can run anaerobically for about 300 yards, so that's the farthest away from the finish line that you should launch your sprint. If you've started the race too fast and have slowed during the second half of the race, you're going to have a tough time kicking for more than 50 to 100 yards.

Track Talk
Your finishing sprint in the last few hundred yards of a race is your **kick**.

The Least You Need to Do

Following are two training schedules, one for building up to a 5K and one for building up to an 8K or 10K. Here's the fine print on these schedules:

➤ They assume that you can manage the first week's training. If you're not at that level yet, build your mileage until you are.

➤ I've only listed the key workouts for each week. Try to get in at least one or two other easy runs at your usual distance during the week.

➤ Don't run so much or so hard the rest of the week that you can't complete the listed workouts. They are the ones that will spur your improvement.

➤ Space the key workouts evenly throughout each week to allow proper recovery.

➤ Try not to miss any of the key workouts, but don't try to "make up" missed ones. Just keep going through the schedule.

➤ If you miss the key workouts two weeks in a row, postpone your goal race by two weeks, and pick up the schedule where you left off.

➤ Do the striders at the end of an easy run. Try not to do them the day after the speed workouts or the long runs.

➤ The speed workouts are in terms of meters. If you don't want to run speed work on the track, translate miles to minutes, and do the workouts on the road or trail.

Training Tip
During your recovery between intervals, keep moving rather than standing bent over. Moving around helps to clear some of the waste products that built up when you were running hard, so you'll be more ready for the next interval. Jog slowly or at least walk.

Rules of the Road
When should you not complete a speed workout? Stop immediately if you have sharp pain anywhere below your waist. Also, if you do the first half of a workout and are running 15 seconds or more slower per mile than usual and there's no obvious reason why, such as bad weather, you're probably overly fatigued from your training.

➤ The schedules include races before your goal race. Enter these to get used to what racing feels like.

➤ Don't run to exhaustion within five days of your goal race.

The speed workouts are in runner shorthand, specifying the number, distance, and pace for the workout. For example, 4×800 meters at 5K goal pace means to do four intervals of 800 meters each at your per mile goal pace for 5K, with the proper recovery between the intervals. Remember, a standard outdoor track is 400 meters around, so 800 meters equals two laps. Also, keep in mind that a 8K/10K goal pace is 10–15 seconds per mile slower than a 5K race pace. Finally, before starting these training schedules, your minimum weekly mileage should be 15 miles for the 5K and 25 miles for the 8K or 10K.

Eight-Week 5K Training Schedule

		Long run	Striders	Speed workout
Week 1	4 miles	8 to 12	4×800 meters	At 10 seconds slower per mile than 5K goal pace
Week 2	5 miles	8 to 12	4×800 meters	At 5K goal pace
Week 3	5 miles	8 to 12	$3 \times 1,200$ meters	At 5K goal pace
Week 4	6 miles	8 to 12	$3 \times 1,600$ meters	At 5 to 10 seconds slower per mile than 5K goal pace
Week 5	6 miles	8 to 12	$3 \times 1,600$ meters	At 5K goal pace
Week 6		8 to 12		5K practice race
Week 7	5 miles	8 to 12	$2 \times 1,600$ meters	At 5 to 10 seconds slower per mile than 5K goal pace
Week 8		8		Goal 5K race

Eight-Week 8K/10K Training Schedule

		Long run	Striders	Speed workout
Week 1	5 miles	8 to 12	4 × 800 meters	At 5K race pace
Week 2	6 miles	8 to 12	3 × 1,200 meters	At 8K/10K goal pace
Week 3	7 miles	8 to 12	3 × 1,200 meters	At 5K race pace
Week 4	8 miles	8 to 12	3 × 1,600 meters	At 8K/10K goal pace
Week 5	8 miles	8 to 12	2 × 2,000 meters	At 8K/10K goal pace
Week 6		8 to 12		At 5K practice pace
Week 7	6 miles	8 to 12	3 × 1,600 meters	At 5K race pace
Week 8		8		Goal 8K/10K race

The Least You Need to Know

➤ To race your best, pick a target distance, and do workouts relevant to the demands of that distance.

➤ The most important aspect of running a faster 5K or 10K is boosting your VO₂ max.

➤ Speed workouts at about your 5K race pace are the best way to improve your VO₂ max.

➤ If you start 5Ks and 10Ks by running faster than your race pace, you'll have to slow dramatically in the second half of the race.

➤ The best race plan is to run an even pace until near the end, then kick to the finish.

Chapter 21

Middle Ground: 15Ks to Half-Marathons

In This Chapter

➤ Why more runners should consider 15Ks and half-marathons

➤ What your lactate threshold is and why it matters

➤ A 10-week training schedule for 15K and half-marathon races

Back when I tried to win the Boston Marathon every year, an important part of my preparation involved a trip to Washington, DC. No, it wasn't so that I could ask President Carter to deny the visas of foreign runners who I thought might beat me. I went there to run the Cherry Blossom 10-miler two weeks before the Boston Marathon to get a good gauge of my race fitness.

Now that I don't race the marathon any more, races of 10 miles or more have become my marathons. They're the longest races I run in a year, and I build up to them like I used to prepare for marathons. Most people don't run these distances. They focus on the extremes—they want to see whether they're fast enough for a 5K or strong enough for a marathon. In this chapter, I'll show you why I think more runners should strike this middle ground of 15Ks and half-marathons, and I'll show you how to train for these races.

The Rodney Dangerfields of Races

Races of 15K (9.3 miles) through the half-marathon (13.1 miles) get no respect. The half-marathon doesn't even get its own name; it's just half of another distance. Imagine if people called 5Ks "half-10Ks."

Track Talk

Tune-up races are shorter races that you use as part of your training for a longer race. Marathoners tune up with 10-milers, 10K runners tune up with 5Ks, and 5K runners tune up with one-mile races.

This range of races, which also includes 10-milers and 20K (12.4 miles), is almost never the focus of a runner's races. Runners usually use these races as *tune-up races* a month or so before a marathon. Or some runners will run one of these races at the beginning of a racing season to build strength, and then drop down in distance to 5Ks and 10Ks for the rest of the season. But you almost never hear a runner say, "This fall, my goal is to be the best 10-mile runner I can be."

That's too bad. These hybrid distances can be some of the most satisfying in running. They're plenty long, so you're not going to get through one by running a few miles a few times a week, as you could with a 5K. But they're not so long that they're going to knock you down for too long. Most of the soreness and lingering fatigue that people have from marathons comes from what happens after 18 or 20 miles.

Footnotes

The fastest times for distances from road races are officially called world bests, rather than world records, because of the great variation among road race courses. When this book went to press, the men's and women's world bests for 10 miles were 44:45, by Paul Koech of Kenya, and 51:39, by Rose Cheruiyot of Kenya. That's 4:28 per mile for Koech and 5:10 per mile for Cheruiyot.

Should you try a 15K, 10-miler, or a half-marathon? Why not? For people who are thinking about trying a marathon someday, building up to one of these races is a good idea. You learn the routine of training for longer distances by gradually extending your distance. Anyone running a marathon should have experience with other races first. These longer races will give you a better idea of what you're going to experience if you try to tackle a marathon.

If you usually don't run farther than five miles, keying on one of these races is a good motivation to extend your distance. In this case, ignore the training schedule at the end of this chapter and make finishing the distance respectably your goal the first time around. To do that, increase the distance of your long run by one mile two out of every three weeks. For 15Ks and 10-milers, work up to running that far two weeks before the race. Take it easy for the next two weeks, and then run the race at a strong but reasonable pace that you know you can maintain to the end. If you're going to do a half-marathon, then build up to 10 to 12 miles at a time, again doing your last long run two weeks before the race.

But if you've been running a bit more and think that you can not only cover the distance, but also run a good notch faster than on your usual training runs, you can improve your performance at these distances by entering the strange world of the lactate threshold.

Beyond the Lactate Threshold

Put on your lab coats: It's time for a little science lesson. As you know by this point in the book, glycogen, a form of stored carbohydrate, is your body's preferred source of fuel for aerobic exercise. The faster you run, the more glycogen your body burns compared to how much fat it burns. Like any chemical burning process, the process of burning glycogen generates by-products. Burn paper, and you get smoke. Burn glycogen, and you get lactate. Lactate is the by-product of your body burning carbohydrates.

You've probably heard about lactic acid. For our purposes here, that's the same thing as lactate. Have you ever tried to sprint all-out for more than a few hundred yards? Remember how at the end of the sprint your muscles felt as though they were on fire? That's because there was a lot of lactate circulating in your system from all the carbohydrates that were suddenly being burned to power you down the track. So much lactate was being produced that your body couldn't clear it from your blood, so your muscles stung.

Some people think that you're damaging your muscles when you expose them to lactate. That's wrong. You're always producing lactate—when you're running easy, when you're walking, even when you're sitting. When you burn carbohydrates, as you almost always do, you produce lactate. Your muscles don't ache at these low levels of effort because the rate of lactate entering your blood is equal to the rate at which it's removed.

As you move up the intensity scale from walking to easy running, you produce more lactate, but your body also increases the rate at which it removes lactate from your blood. When you exercise above a certain intensity, however, the rate at which you produce lactate is greater than the rate at which your body can clear it. The lactate concentration rises in your muscles and blood, and suddenly your effort feels much harder. At this point, you've reached your *lactate threshold*.

You're probably thinking, "Thanks for the biochemistry lesson, but what does this have to do with running a 10-mile race?" Remember the basic race-training

Track Talk
The exercise intensity at which you produce more lactate than your body can remove is your *lactate threshold*. Having a high lactate threshold means that you can maintain a faster pace for a longer distance before you have to slow. An experienced runner's lactate threshold is approximately his or her 15K to half-marathon race pace.

principle that I laid down last chapter: If you want to complete a race, you have to be able to cover the distance. If you also want to *race* the distance, then you should do workouts that improve your capacities to handle the limiting factors on your performance in that distance. For 5Ks and 10Ks, that meant doing workouts to max out your VO_2 max. For 15Ks to half-marathons, that means improving your lactate threshold.

Once you get past the hump of being able to cover the distance without great fatigue, the limiting factor on how fast you can run the 15K to the half-marathon is your lactate threshold. In fact, your race pace for the 15K to the half-marathon is roughly equal to your lactate threshold. Go faster than that, and you'll start accumulating lactate in your blood. You can exceed your lactate threshold in shorter races, such as an 8K, but 15Ks to half-marathons last one to two hours for most runners, and you just can't run that fast for that long.

To improve, then, you need to increase your lactate threshold. When you do that, your lactate threshold occurs at a higher percentage of your VO_2 max. So with the right training, you can push your 15K to half-marathon pace closer to that of your 5K pace; that is, you can make better use of your basic aerobic fitness. You can run faster before you start accumulating lactate.

Timing Is Everything: All About Tempo Runs

Improving your lactate threshold is pretty straightforward: You train at or slightly above your lactate threshold. In the training schedule, I call this speed your LT (lactate threshold) pace. Training at your LT pace pushes back the point at which lactate accumulates, allowing you to maintain a faster pace for these mid-range races.

How do you know what this pace is for you? If you already race in 15K to half-marathons, your race pace for those races is your LT pace. If you haven't raced much, you can still approximate what your LT pace is. If you've run a 10K, your LT pace will be about 20 seconds slower per mile than your 10K race pace. If you've only run a 5K, your LT pace is probably around 30 seconds slower per mile than your 5K race pace is, but you should go run a 10K first anyway before trying to race a 15K to half-marathon.

Training Tip

A good way to know if you're at the right intensity during an LT run is a modified version of the talk test. You should be able to say a few words coherently at a normal conversational speed. If you can only blurt out a word at a time, you're going too fast. If you can speak in complete sentences, you're going too slow.

Regardless of what pace you choose to shoot for, keep this guideline in mind: Your effort during LT workouts should feel "comfortably hard." You should feel as though you're working at a high level that you can sustain. If you were to increase your pace by 10 seconds or more per mile, you would have to slow within a few minutes.

It's important to run as close to the right pace for as much of your LT workouts as possible. Remember what I told you in the last chapter about training to improve your VO_2 max:

The biggest gains come from doing the workout in that small window where you're most stressing the systems that you want to improve.

When you do LT workouts, you'll probably think in the first mile that you should be going faster. After all, you're not all that much out of breath. Stick to your pace. The point of the workout is to run it all at your LT pace. That's different than starting out too fast, and then slowing in the second half of your LT workout. In that case, you might average the right pace for the whole workout, but never run any part of it at the right intensity. That kind of workout won't improve your LT as much.

The classic workout to improve your lactate threshold is the *tempo run*, a continuous run of 20 to 40 minutes at LT pace. An example of a tempo run workout is a two-mile warm-up, a four-mile run at your LT pace, and a short cool-down jog. You can also do LT intervals. In these workouts, you do two or three intervals of a fairly long distance at LT pace, jog easily for 25 to 50 percent of the duration of the interval, and then repeat the sequence. For example, after warming up, you would run two miles at your LT pace, jog for five minutes, run two miles at your LT pace, and then do a cool-down jog.

Track Talk
A *tempo run* is a run of 20 to 40 minutes at about your 15K to half-marathon race pace. It builds your ability to sustain a hard pace for a long time.

In the training schedule, I start you with LT intervals to get you used to the workouts and to help you learn what your LT pace feels like. Once you're familiar with your LT pace, I have you do tempo runs. Tempo runs are better because you become more accustomed to concentrating for an extended period while you're running hard. This kind of training helps you mentally in your races.

Training Tip
If you do your tempo runs with someone else, take turns sharing the lead. Switch positions every mile.

At first, you should do LT workouts on the track or other accurately measured courses so that you have a way of checking your pace. After a few LT workouts, you should have a feel for the pace. Studies have shown that most runners can accurately produce that "comfortably hard" level of effort on their own once they have learned it. This frees you to do your LT workouts on the roads or trails. Doing a five-mile tempo run on the track can get pretty boring, after all. Doing some of your LT workouts away from the track is an especially good idea if you'll be running a hilly race because you'll be more used to running LT pace over a variety of terrain.

Not many runners know about these workouts. They think that to run a faster half-marathon, they should work on their speed, so they run 800-meter intervals. This type of workout does make them faster, but it doesn't do much for their ability to sustain a pretty hard pace for more than an hour.

Training Tip
If you're sore the day after a tempo run, then you ran it too fast.

Those who do talk about doing tempo training throw around the words pretty haphazardly. They'll say they're doing an "uptempo run," when all they mean is that they're going to go a little harder than usual for a few miles in the middle of a run. Or they'll go out and run a hard 10 miles and say that's their tempo run for the week. They can call it whatever they want, but these aren't really tempo runs. Unlike you, they don't know why they should do these 20- to 40-minute runs at a precise pace.

Why didn't I include tempo runs in Chapter 19 when I talked about various types of workouts? Because those were workouts that I think all runners should do some version of. LT workouts are only necessary if you're going to be doing races of 15K or longer. Then they make an incredible difference in your performance. Besides, I didn't want to let everyone in on our little secret.

The Least You Need to Do

Before starting this training schedule, be sure to review the long list of training advice that I gave before the training schedules in the last chapter. Everything I said there about how to structure your training weeks for 5K and 10K races applies here, too. Here are some additional guidelines for races of 15K to the half-marathon:

➤ The schedule assumes that your weekly mileage is at 30 miles when you begin the schedule.

➤ The schedule assumes that you have already completed a 15K to half-marathon race and now want to improve your time.

➤ The schedule assumes that you have run a 5K to 10K race within a few months of starting the schedule so that you have a way of setting a 15K/half-marathon goal pace. Remember that your LT pace is equal to your goal pace for the 15K/half-marathon, 20 seconds per mile slower than your 10K race pace, or 30 seconds per mile slower than your 5K race pace.

➤ The schedule assumes that you can complete the first week of training without it killing you.

➤ You run two workouts in the schedule faster than LT pace. You'll run these workouts at fairly close to 10K race pace. These workouts will help to improve your VO_2 max, which is also important for racing a good 15K or half-marathon.

➤ The schedule includes two tune-up races, the first either a 5K or 8K and the second either an 8K or 10K. These races will also improve your VO_2 max. Use these races to practice your race routine and to monitor your progress. Don't worry if your 5K time isn't what you think it should be. The focus of your training is on improving your lactate threshold, not your VO_2 max.

➤ On race day, warm up with half a mile to a mile of easy jogging and a few striders at LT pace to remind yourself what the pace feels like. Finish your warm-up no more than 10 minutes before the start, and then keep moving to keep your heart rate elevated.

➤ Run as even a pace as you can in your race. Starting too quickly will push you beyond your lactate threshold and not allow you to use your training. From the start of the race, try to get in that pace that you've run so many times in your workouts.

> **Rules of the Road**
> Be sure to drink plenty of fluids during your 15K to half-marathon races. You're going to be out there for more than an hour and can get dehydrated easily.

After your race, run easily for one to two weeks, and then pick a new goal to start working toward.

Ten-Week 15K/Half-Marathon Training Schedule

	Long run	Striders	Speed workout
Week 1	8 miles	8 to 12	2 × 3,200 meters at LT pace
Week 2	10 miles	8 to 12	2 × 4,000 meters at LT pace
Week 3	12 miles	8 to 12	6,400 meters (4 miles) at LT pace
Week 4		8 to 12	4 × 1,600 meters at 15 seconds per mile faster than LT pace
Week 5	13 miles	8 to 12	8,000 meters (5 miles) at LT pace
Week 6		8 to 12	5K or 8K practice race
Week 7	15 miles	8 to 12	8,000 meters (5 miles) at LT pace
Week 8		8 to 12	8K or 10K practice race
Week 9	10 miles	8 to 12	3 × 1,600 meters at 15 seconds per mile faster than LT pace
Week 10		8	Goal 15K or half-marathon race

Footnotes

At the 1994 Gasparilla 15K, elite runners Jon Brown and Phillimon Hanneck were assigned a room together for race weekend. On race day, Hanneck discovered that he had packed only one racing shoe. Brown lent one of his extras to Hanneck, even though Brown's foot was several sizes larger. Hanneck repaid the favor by narrowly edging Brown for the victory.

The Least You Need to Know

➤ More runners should consider doing races in the 15K to half-marathon range.

➤ If you haven't run one of these races before, run one to complete it before you try to race it.

➤ Your lactate threshold is the pace at which you begin to accumulate lactic acid in your blood.

➤ When you race a 15K to half-marathon, you're running at your lactate threshold.

➤ The best way to improve your performance in 15K to half-marathon races is to improve your lactate threshold.

➤ The best way to improve your lactate threshold is to do runs of 20 to 40 minutes at your lactate threshold pace.

Chapter 22

In It for the Long Run: The Marathon

In This Chapter

➤ History of the marathon

➤ Deciding whether the marathon is right for you

➤ How to train for your first marathon

The marathon is the crown jewel of running. Some have called it the ultimate race. I made it the focus of my running—OK, the focus of my life—for 15 years. The challenge of running 26.2 miles is something that no other race can provide.

You can't roll out of bed and run a marathon. Finishing one is a lot of hard work, not just during the race, but in all those miles you log just to get to the starting line. And yet, almost anyone can finish a marathon. Grandmothers do it; cancer patients do it; even Oprah Winfrey and the Vice President of the United States have done it. It's not easy, but it's simple. In this chapter, I'll show you the basic training that you need to complete if you want to proudly wear those crown jewels.

A Little History

I told you before about how your body can usually store only enough glycogen to fuel about 20 miles of running. And yet marathons are 26.2 miles long. What gives?

The legend of the origin of the marathon goes like this: In 490 B.C., a Greek messenger named Pheidippides ran the 24 miles from the Plains of Marathon to Athens to announce that despite great odds, the Athenian army had defeated the invading Persians. Upon reaching Athens, Pheidippides said, "Rejoice. We conquer!" collapsed, and died. When the modern Olympics began in Athens in 1896, organizers included a 24-mile race from Marathon to Athens to honor this great moment in Greek history.

Footnotes

When this book went to press, the men's and women's world marathon bests were 2:06:50, by Belayneh Densimo of Ethiopia, and 2:21:06, by Ingrid Kristiansen of Norway. That's 4:50 per mile for Densimo and 5:22 per mile for Kristiansen.

Did this really happen? No one knows for sure, but the general consensus is that like any good story from antiquity, there's some embellishment stirred in to the truth so well that it's hard to separate the two, and it's more fun not to bother anyway. There was a Greek messenger of the time named Pheidippides, but no contemporary record of him producing such a great deathbed quote exists. Nonetheless, the legend has its own resonance. At the 20-mile mark of his first marathon, Frank Shorter turned to a runner next to him and said, "Why couldn't have Pheidippides have died at 20 miles?"

The long race caught on after the 1896 Olympics. The first Boston Marathon was held the next year. Early marathons weren't standardized—they were 24 or 25 miles, depending on how long a course turned out to be. Early in this century, the starting line of a marathon in England was moved back so that the Queen could watch from Windsor Castle. The resulting distance was 26 miles, 385 yards, or 26.2 miles, which is now the official distance for a marathon.

Is This Really Necessary?

The marathon is one of the greatest challenges in sports. That's why so many runners are drawn to it. Run a marathon, and you know that you've really accomplished something.

Some runners think that they have to run a marathon to become a "real runner." They think that no one will think they're legitimate runners otherwise. That's not true. No one is less of a runner for not running a marathon. I don't race marathons any more, but someone must still think I'm OK because I got to write this book. One of the most revered figures in American running, Steve Prefontaine, never ran a marathon. And if how far you run in a race determines your worthiness as a runner, then shouldn't we all be aiming for 50-milers, 100-milers, or even the six-day races that a few runners do?

Footnotes

The American record for the marathon for women is 2:21:21 by Joan Benoit Samuelson. What counts as the American marathon record for men is a source of confusion because some courses, such as the Boston Marathon, aren't officially allowed for record purposes. (The Boston Marathon course doesn't count for record purposes because there's too much of a net elevation drop on its point-to-point course.) The official American marathon record for men is 2:09:35 by Jerry Lawson, set at the Chicago Marathon. The recognized American best is 2:08:47 by Bob Kempainen, set at the Boston Marathon.

Training for and running a marathon takes a lot of work. When the going gets tough, you're going to come face to face with your soul, and you're going to ask, "Why am I doing this?" Before doing a marathon, you should be able to answer that question with your own reasons, not someone else's standards.

Caveat Runner

Even if you're all fired up to run a marathon for all the right reasons, you have to tread carefully. You're going to be doing training runs that are substantially longer than anything you've ever done. If you don't become an expert at listening to your body's response to the training, you might not even make it to the starting line. It's not uncommon for runners to have to postpone or give up their marathon hopes because the training necessary to do one is too much for their current level of fitness.

I think you should be a regular runner for at least a year before starting to train for a marathon. You need that amount of time for basic strength building to get your muscles, tendons, bones, and ligaments used to the stress of running. You also need to be in a good training routine, having figured out how best to make your running work with the rest of your life.

Footnotes

The great Czech runner Emil Zatopek ran his first marathon in the 1952 Olympics. Unsure how to pace himself, he ran with the world record holder, Jim Peters of Great Britain. After 10 miles, Zatopek asked Peters, "The pace, Jim, it is too fast?" Peters wanted to toy with Zatopek and trick him into burning himself out, so he coyly replied, "No, Emil. The pace, it is too slow." Zatopek took off and never looked back, winning the Olympic Marathon in his first attempt at the distance!

Don't even think about starting to train for a marathon if you're injured. Doing the long runs that are necessary to finish a marathon is exactly the kind of repetitive stress that will make your injury even worse. But if you want to run a marathon for yourself, and if you've been running regularly for at least a year, and if you're currently running injury-free, then let's get going!

A Run or a Race?

The fastest male marathoners in the world run 26.2 miles at faster than 5:00 per mile. The fastest female marathoners in the world run 26.2 miles at faster than 5:30 per mile. I think we can safely say that these people are racing the marathon. That was certainly how I went about it. For me, the challenge wasn't just running 26.2 miles; it was seeing how fast I could run 26.2 miles. When I ran marathons at 5:00 per mile, I was running about a minute faster per mile than my usual training pace.

Footnotes

I have the world record for the most marathons run faster than 2:15. I've done that 28 times.

Most people, however, are running the marathon just to conquer the distance. I'm all in favor of that approach. Remember the basic principle from Chapter 20: The first step to participating in any race is being able to cover the distance. The longer the race, the more that negotiating the distance becomes a limiting factor in performance. Almost anyone can run one mile faster than their regular training pace. Almost no one can run 50 miles faster than their regular training pace.

For your first marathon, your goal should be to finish. Trust me, that's more than enough challenge for one race. If you define a race as trying to run the best that you can for a set distance on a given day, then just finishing your first marathon is a race. After you've done one or two marathons, then you can try to reduce your time.

Don't Hit The Wall

You might hear a runner explaining why she dropped out of a 5K by saying, "I hit The Wall." Well, now she's got two strikes against her: Not only did she not finish her race, but she's misusing runner lingo. Get her a copy of this book and quick! When you get tired in a short race because you're breathing so hard, that's fatigue. When you're doing a run of 90 minutes or more, and you're feeling fine, and then all of a sudden, bam, every step is a major production and your pace gets way slower, that's *The Wall*.

Most people can store enough glycogen in their muscles to fuel about 18 to 20 miles of running. When you run long distances, your body senses that it's getting low on glycogen. It wants to preserve that glycogen, so it starts to burn more fat. At this point, you're able to maintain your pace, so you keep running. Your body has to keep doling out its precious glycogen stores, and it starts burning more and more fat.

By now, you can keep up your pace, but you have to work a little harder to do so because fat doesn't burn as efficiently as glycogen when it comes to fueling your running. But you keep running because you were idiotic enough to listen to me when I told you how great the marathon is. Now your glycogen stores are getting very low, and you're burning more and more fat.

That wouldn't be all bad, except for this fact: Fat burns on a flame of glycogen. To keep running at your normal pace, you need at least enough glycogen to help burn the fat. But you've pretty much used it all up. You're primarily burning fat, and fat takes a lot more oxygen to burn than glycogen does. As a result, you have to slow down dramatically, sometimes by more than two minutes per mile. You will want nothing more than to lie down by the side of the road.

To top it off, you've also depleted the small amount of glycogen that's stored in your liver. Your liver is supposed to feed this glycogen into your bloodstream to maintain your blood sugar well enough to feed your brain glucose. When this process starts breaking down, you feel woozy, light-headed, uncoordinated. Great! You want to lie down by the side of the road, and now you're getting so uncoordinated that you just might have your wish fulfilled. You've got as many as eight miles to go. Unless you've got incredible willpower, you're a leading candidate to join the *DNF* list.

So how do people ever survive marathons? First and most important, they train. Long runs improve your body's ability to store glycogen. Runners who do marathon training can store more than twice as much glycogen in their muscles as untrained people. Your body can get more fuel from the food that you eat when you train properly.

Track Talk
When you've run so far that you've depleted your muscles' glycogen stores, you hit *The Wall*. Most runners crash into it at about the 20-mile mark of the marathon.

Track Talk
If you did not finish a race, you're a *DNF*. DNF is also a verb, as in, "How did you do?" "I DNFed."

Training Tip
Do your long runs at your normal training pace. A good habit is to do the second half of your run 10 seconds per mile faster than the first half. This strategy helps you to start the run slow enough so that you'll be able to finish it, and picking up the pace a bit at the end teaches you how to concentrate when you get tired.

Also, marathoners start their marathons at a pace they know that they can maintain to the finish. The faster you run, the more glycogen you burn. Going out too fast in a marathon is a huge mistake, because even at a reasonable pace you're going to need every last bit of glycogen that you can get. One trick that runners do to make sure that they don't go out too fast in the marathon is to run the first mile one minute slower than the pace that they hope to average for the distance.

Even if you do the right training and pace yourself well in the marathon, The Wall can be pretty daunting. But what you do in the few days before the marathon can push it past the finish line.

The Rest Is Easy

If you look closely at the training schedules in the two previous chapters, you might have noticed that I have you doing less work as your goal race nears, not more. That's especially the case in the marathon schedule—your last long run is three weeks before your marathon. Whatever happened to use it or lose it?

Track Talk
When you cut back on your training before an important race, you're *tapering*. This reduction in training allows your muscles to be able to perform on race day.

Preparing for a top effort isn't like cramming for a test or meeting a deadline at work. It takes time for your body to get the benefits of a training session. The day after a long run, you feel tired. But two weeks later, you feel stronger. The longer your race, the more important *tapering* is.

In the marathon, tapering is especially important because of the whole glycogen-storage issue. When you taper, then obviously you're not draining your glycogen supply as much. But because of your long runs, you've tricked your muscles into thinking that they had better be ready anytime, anywhere to fuel you for hours. So even though you're barely running, they're still suspicious that something is up, and they keep stockpiling glycogen at a high level. This gives you a larger gas tank on race day.

Rules of the Road
Postpone your marathon if in the last two weeks before it you develop a cold that lasts for more than three days. Your immune system is depressed after a marathon anyway, so the two things together could really knock you back.

Notice what I said—you're barely running. That's a lot different than not running at all. If you follow the tapering plan in the marathon schedule, you'll maintain the benefits of your hard work. Once you become fit, you don't have to do as much running to maintain that fitness, at least for awhile. So in the three weeks before your marathon, you can, and should, gradually reduce your training.

Do your longest run three weeks before the marathon. The following week, do no more than 75 percent of your usual weekly mileage. The week after that, do no more than 60 percent of your usual weekly mileage. And the week before the marathon, do no more than 50 percent of your usual weekly mileage.

Spaghetti for Dinner Again?

In Chapter 13, I told you that eating isn't the key to running well. That's true. A good diet merely allows you to get the most from your running; it doesn't take the place of running. But I also told you that there's nothing you can eat to make you a better runner.

Confession time: That's not entirely true. In the few days before a marathon, you can help to push The Wall a few more miles back by *carboloading*.

Carboloading is often misunderstood. It doesn't mean looking at the last three days before a marathon as an excuse to hit every all-you-can-eat buffet in town. You're running less; you don't need to eat much more than you usually do. What matters is increasing the percentage of your calories that come from carbohydrates to more than 65 percent, not just chowing down on everything in sight.

Carboloading works for the same reason that tapering works. Your muscles have become trained to store more glycogen. You're tapering, so you're not running much. Good—you're barely dipping into your fuel stores. Simultaneously, you're eating more carbohydrates than usual. Your muscles love it! They soak up the stuff. Do it right, and you can store an additional few hundred calories. That's worth an extra three miles of running!

The key to carboloading is to emphasize the right foods. Concentrate on basing all of your meals in the three days before a marathon on high-carb foods, especially the complex ones. Most runners eat pasta when they're carboloading, but rice and other grains are good, too. As I pointed out in Chapter 13, be sure that what you think is high-carb really is. Fettucini alfredo is pasta, but it's pasta in a heavy cream sauce. If you're going to eat pasta, go with the light red sauces.

Track Talk
Increasing the percentage of your calories that comes from carbohydrates to more than 65 percent in the few days before a long race is *carboloading*.

Training Tip
If you can, avoid the spaghetti feeds held the night before marathons. You'll use up a lot of mental energy at these loud, boisterous affairs. Have your pre-race dinner in a quiet setting with family and friends. You'll have several hours the next day to spend with the runners.

The Least You Need to Do

To finish a marathon, the least you need to do is still pretty darned much. There's no way to get around the necessity of long runs—that's why they're the focus of this marathon training schedule. As a first-time marathoner, your goal should be to cover the distance. The way to do that is to gradually build the distance that you can cover without having to slow dramatically in the last few miles.

These long runs are probably longer than you've ever run. They're all the training stress that your body needs, so this schedule doesn't include any speed workouts. At this point, they'll just get in the way of recovering from your long runs. But you will be doing striders. Most weeks, you'll be doing them twice. That's because when you do nothing but train for marathons, it's easy for your form to deteriorate. You're always just shuffling along, not moving through a full range of motion. Striders will help you to improve your form, and they're a fun contrast to the long runs.

Where the schedule says "2 × 12" under striders, that means that on two other runs that week, do striders. When it says "1 × 12," just do striders once that week. Make one of your striders days the last run that you do before the next week's long run. For example, if your long run is on a Sunday and you are going for a run the previous Friday, do striders on Friday. Don't do striders the day after a long run.

The schedule doesn't have you running a long run every week. That would be too much because your long run starts getting up there in distance. On the weeks when you're not going long, you'll see that it says "10 miles" under the "Hilly run" column heading. On these weeks, I want you to do a hilly 10-mile run on the day that you usually do your long run. This run will help to build leg strength and will give your VO_2 max a bit of a boost.

The long runs are the key to this schedule. How much you run the rest of the week depends on how quickly you recover from the long runs. You should be running at least two other days most weeks. (Gotta do those striders!) It would be good if most weeks you included a run in the middle of the week that was half the distance of your last long run.

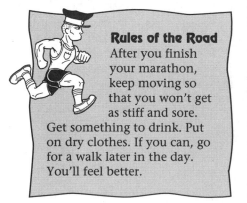

Rules of the Road
After you finish your marathon, keep moving so that you won't get as stiff and sore. Get something to drink. Put on dry clothes. If you can, go for a walk later in the day. You'll feel better.

For example, in week 6, your last long run was an 18-miler in week 5. So in week 6, do a 9-miler in addition to the hilly 10-miler. These medium-long runs in the middle of the week will help to consolidate the gains from the long run.

With two weeks to go, try to run a 15K to half-marathon race. Don't worry so much about your pace as about experiencing a race atmosphere. A lot of first-time marathoners train in isolation for months, never enter a race, and freak out when suddenly they're surrounded by thousands of others in a marathon.

As with the training schedules in the previous two chapters, this one assumes that you can handle the first week's training. If you've gone on a 12-mile run within the last two weeks, you can. If you haven't, take your time building up to that level, and then report back when you're ready.

Twelve-Week Training Schedule for First-Time Marathoners

	Long run	Striders	Hilly run
Week 1	14 miles	2×12	
Week 2	15 miles	2×12	
Week 3	16 miles	2×12	
Week 4		2×12	10 miles
Week 5	18 miles	2×12	
Week 6		2×12	10 miles
Week 7	20 miles	2×12	
Week 8		2×12	10 miles
Week 9	20 to 22 miles	2×12	
Week 10	15K or half-marathon practice race	1×12	
Week 11	10 miles	2×12	
Week 12	Marathon	6	

The Least You Need to Know

➤ You don't have to run a marathon to consider yourself a runner.

➤ Your goal in your first marathon should be to finish.

➤ The key to finishing a marathon is building your weekly long run to at least 20 miles.

➤ Training, tapering, and carboloading help you to avoid hitting The Wall.

My Favorite Races

Every year, more than 10,000 road races are held in the United States alone. From big-city mega races, such as the New York City Marathon, to intimate club races among a handful of hard-core runners, to all distances and sizes between, races of all types are held every weekend.

I've run in every kind of race there is. (In fact, some days my legs feel as if I've run in every race ever held.) Every race I've run has had something special about it, and if I look back in my training log and see some race that I ran 10 years ago, I can usually remember the course, the people, and so on just like a lot of baseball pitchers say they can remember every pitch they've ever thrown. But some races stand out above the rest. Maybe it's the course or the race's history or its purpose—whatever it is, these races have something that makes me put a mental asterisk next to them. In this chapter, I'll tell you what my favorite races are and why.

Bill's Top 10 List

Every year, I go to more than 30 races. Multiply that by 30 years of running, and you can see that I just plain like to be at the races. So having to limit myself to naming my 10 favorite races is as constraining as having to list my 10 favorite foods. But if David Letterman can come up with a top 10 list every night, surely I can manage just this once.

Without further adieu, here are my 10 favorite races:

➤ The Boston Marathon

➤ The New York City Marathon

➤ The Falmouth Road Race

➤ The Bix 7-Miler

➤ The Walt Disney World Marathon

➤ Any Thanksgiving race

➤ My Jingle Bell Runs

➤ The Race for the Cure Series

➤ The Chase Corporate Challenge Series

➤ The Avon Mini Marathon

I have a point in listing something as vague as "any Thanksgiving race." You'll see why as you read what I think is special about the races on my top 10 list.

The Boston Marathon

If you've heard of one runner's race, this is probably it. I'll make you a bet: Within your first year of running, if enough people see you running, eventually one of them is going to ask you, "Whaddya trainin' for the Boston Marathon?" Another prediction: If you start going to races and let others know about it, eventually one of them will ask, "So, have you run the Boston Marathon?" There's no more famous race in the world.

Just the Facts

The Boston Marathon starts at noon on Patriot's Day every year. Patriot's Day is a New England holiday that commemorates the Battle of Lexington on April 19, 1775; in Massachusetts, it's a state holiday, and it falls on the third Monday in April. The race begins in Hopkinton, Massachusetts and ends in downtown Boston. The Boston Marathon is put on by the Boston Athletic Association. For an application, write BAA Boston Marathon, The Starting Line, One Ash Street, Hopkinton, MA 01748-1897; or visit the Web site, http://www.boston-marathon.org.

What's So Special About Boston?

The Boston Marathon has it all: more than a century of history, a great course, and spectacular spectators. For average runners, it's unique among marathons in that it has qualifying standards. The standards were introduced in 1971 to make the size of the field more manageable. The qualifying time has to be run on an accurately measured course within just more than a year before the Boston Marathon that you want to participate in. The current standards are shown in the following list:

Age Group	Men	Women
18 to 34	3:10	3:40
35 to 39	3:15	3:45
40 to 44	3:20	3:50
45 to 49	3:25	3:55
50 to 54	3:30	4:00
55 to 59	3:35	4:05
60 to 64	3:40	4:10
65 to 69	3:45	4:15
70+	3:50	4:20

These standards are tough! For example, if you're a woman under the age of 35, you have to run 26.2 miles at an average pace of 8:25 per mile or faster. Older folks certainly don't get a break: a 70-year-old man has to average about 8:45 a mile for 26.2 miles just to make it to Boston's starting line.

But rather than resent these standards, most runners I know appreciate them. After a few years of running, a lot of runners look at qualifying for Boston as their personal Olympics. Even if they make it just once in their lives, or even if they fall short, they value the challenge that the Boston qualifying standards offer. If only for this once in their running life, they like the idea of having this inflexible goal that they're willing to make great sacrifices to meet.

Footnotes

The first Boston Marathon was held in 1897. Most people call it the oldest continually held marathon in the world. Purists point out that in 1918, the usual marathon was replaced by a 25-mile relay race among 10-man military teams.

What's so special about Boston? Pretty much everything. Sure, I'm a bit biased. Winning Boston in 1975 was the first major victory of my career, and I was fortunate enough to be able to win three more times by 1980. In two of those wins, I set the course and American best (2:09:55 in 1975, and then 2:09:27 in 1979).

The most special thing about Boston is its course and the crowds that line it. You start in a small, New England village and then make your way through several towns with names that have meaning to all marathoners: Ashland, Framingham, Natick, and so on. Near halfway, you pass an all-women's college, Wellesley, where the roar from the students was so loud that when three-time champion Ibrahim Hussein passed through in 1992, he covered his ears. Then it's the famous Newton Hills, finishing with *Heartbreak Hill*, which crests at 21 miles. From its top, you have five mostly downhill miles to the finish right near Copley Square in downtown Boston.

Footnotes

Heartbreak Hill is probably the most famous hill in running history. It's the last of the four major hills on the Boston Marathon course between 16 and 21 miles. It got its name in 1936 from a writer covering the race for the *Boston Globe*. It was on this hill that year that the defending champion, Johnny A. Kelley, was passed by Tarzan Brown, and then faded to fifth. As hills go, it's not all that tough, but try telling that to your legs 20 miles into a marathon.

Along the way are the greatest crowds in running. When the 100th Boston Marathon was run in 1996, more than two million spectators were on the route. Many of them stake their claim hours before the start at noon to ensure a good viewing spot. You'll see parties and cookouts nearly every mile. So much for the loneliness of the long-distance runner! Running the Boston Marathon gives you an idea what the sport is like in Europe and Japan, where the fans are as numerous and knowledgeable about running as they are here about football.

The New York City Marathon

If you've heard of a marathon besides Boston, it's probably New York. After all, it's kind of hard to ignore 30,000 people running through all five boroughs of the world's most famous city.

Just the Facts

After initially being held in October, the New York City Marathon is now held on the first Sunday in November in an attempt to escape the Indian summer days that often plagued runners during the earlier dates. The race's popularity has continued to soar as it approaches its 30th running in 1999. In 1997, more than 30,000 runners started the race, which was a record field for New York.

The New York City Marathon is the gem of the weekly races put on by the New York Road Runners Club. Because so many people want to run in the New York Marathon, the field is limited by a lottery, with many of the spots saved for overseas runners. To request an application, write Marathon Entries, P.O. Box 1388 GPO, New York, NY 10116; call (212) 423-2249; or visit the Web site, http://www.nyrrc.org.

I Love New York

The New York City Marathon is special to me for many of the same reasons that the Boston Marathon is. Before I made my big breakthrough as a marathoner at Boston in 1975, I dropped out of that race in 1973. When New York was held entirely in Central Park, I ran it and struggled there, too, placing fifth in 1974 in 2:35 after thinking that I could win. So it was sweet to win Boston for the first time in the spring of 1975, and then come back to win the 1976 New York City Marathon after a disappointing run in the Olympic Marathon a few months earlier.

Footnotes

The New York City Marathon began as a five-loop run through Manhattan's Central Park. In 1976, race director Fred Lebow convinced the local authorities that it would be good publicity for the city to run through all five of New York's boroughs. This proved to be such a good idea that within 10 years almost every major city in the United States had its own urban marathon.

Starting in 1976, the race moved to the streets of all of New York's five boroughs. The course has been tweaked a bit since then, but the essence remains the same. You start by crossing the Verrazano Narrows Bridge on Staten Island, and then you go through Queens, Brooklyn, and The Bronx and enter the island of Manhattan on First Avenue, about 17 miles into the race. The last three miles are the toughest because you're in hilly Central Park. The race ends in front of world-famous Tavern on the Green restaurant.

I was able to win three more New York Marathons from 1977 to 1979. In those years, it and the Boston Marathon were the main focus of my training. I'd run Boston in the spring, recover, start my build-up during the summer for New York in the fall, recover from that, and start all over again in the winter for the next Boston. Many runners follow a similar plan. New York and other fall marathons fall at a good time of the year—you can train a lot during the early fall, when the weather won't zap you as much as during the summer, run the marathon, and then spend the rest of the year, when it's dark and cold and you're busy with holidays, recovering.

New York is also special because, as at Boston, the whole city gets behind the race. What else unites New York's famously surly residents in such a way? For the week before the marathon, the city has a special atmosphere that's full of cooperation and goodwill. That feeling carries over to race day, when more than a million people line the streets for hours, cheering. As Olympic champion Frank Shorter said, if you don't get goosebumps when you head up First Avenue, there's something wrong with you.

The Falmouth Road Race

What's that you say? You've always wanted to run a race that starts on an incredibly narrow drawbridge and finishes right next to the Atlantic Ocean? Then look no further than the Falmouth Road Race.

Just the Facts

The Falmouth Road Race is held in the middle of August. It starts in Woods Hole, Massachusetts (site of a famous oceanographic institute and the ferry to Martha's Vineyard) and ends 7.1 miles later in seaside Falmouth. More than 8,000 runners take part every year. For an application, write P.O. Box 732, Falmouth, MA 02541; or call (508) 540-7000.

Ocean Motion

Falmouth is great for several reasons. It embodies the celebratory nature of racing that I'm so fond of; you finish right next to a huge field, where a post-race party/barbecue is held. Although some of the best runners in the world are in the field, the race has a vacation-like feel. I know one runner who makes it his only race of the year; he's just so drawn to the atmosphere of New England by the ocean in late summer. I also like the point-to-point course that builds momentum as you near the finish, like at Boston.

Track Talk

A *course record* is the fastest time run over a given race route. Most races maintain both open course records (the fastest that anyone has run on the course) and age-group course records (for example, the fastest time by a 40-year-old).

Speaking of the course, Falmouth's course is one of the most beautiful in all of road racing. At about two miles, you run past a lighthouse that looks like something out of a Norman Rockwell painting. For most of the race, you're either running along the ocean or on roads through shaded forests. Right at the end, you come over the top of a hill to descend the last few hundred yards to the finish line, where there's always a huge crowd.

I won Falmouth three times outright and have won the master's (age 40-and-over) division there as well. Joan Benoit Samuelson is the only other person to do that. In all, I've set three types of *course records* at Falmouth: in the 20 to 29 division, the 30 to 39 division, and the 40 to 49 division. I hope to do so in the 50 to 59 division this year.

The Bix 7-Miler

Another race that I look forward to every year is the Bix 7-Miler. Like Falmouth, it's a summer race at a nonstandard distance, but that's the least interesting thing about it.

Just the Facts

The Bix 7-Miler, or just Bix, as everyone calls it, is held in late July in Davenport, Iowa. The race was started as part of an annual festival held in honor of Bix Beiderbecke, a seminal jazz trumpeter of the 1920s. Now, with 18,000 entrants, the race has become bigger than any other part of the festival. For more information, write 2685 Kimberly Road, Davenport, IA 52722; or call (319) 324-8657.

Get Your Kicks at Bix

Bix's seven-mile course is a tough one, including a huge hill right off the bat in the first mile. The weather is usually tough, too, what with the race held in the middle of summer in the middle of America's farmland. Conditions at race time in 1997, for example, were 83 degrees with 80 percent humidity. These aren't optimal running conditions!

So what's the big deal about Bix? Why not go somewhere you can run fast? Certainly, running on flat courses where you have a better chance of running a personal best can be fun, but always doing that is boring. If speed is your only goal, why not just go around a track? I think there's more to racing than just seeing how fast you can go. Races that have character, like Bix, are challenging; running them is a good way to test your character as a runner.

Few things are going to get you through a tough course on a tough day any better than the incredibly supportive crowds that the race has. In addition to the great hometown pride of the Quad Cities' residents, you're guaranteed several more thousand spectators thanks to the concurrent jazz festival. I don't mean to sound like I do nothing but party, but this race, too, has a great celebratory atmosphere, including steamboat casinos drifting by on the nearby Mississippi River.

Bix has a strong personal connection for me, too, and not just because I was able to win a couple of times or because, I'm almost embarrassed to note, the city is putting a statue of me along the course. Bix hits home with me because in the 1890s, my relatives owned a house on that big hill in the first mile. Just across the river in Illinois was a family farm. Now when I go to Bix every year with my brother, Charlie, the race has that much more meaning to us.

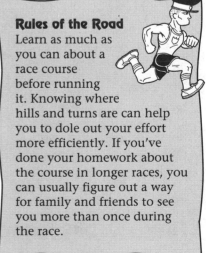

Rules of the Road
Learn as much as you can about a race course before running it. Knowing where hills and turns are can help you to dole out your effort more efficiently. If you've done your homework about the course in longer races, you can usually figure out a way for family and friends to see you more than once during the race.

The Walt Disney World Marathon

Maybe you're starting to think that all of my favorite races are older ones that I've won. Not so. The Walt Disney World Marathon has been around only since the beginning of this decade, and I've never even competed seriously in it, much less won it, but it's still worth recommending.

Just the Facts

The Walt Disney World Marathon is held in early January in, appropriately enough, Walt Disney World or more specifically, Lake Buena Vista, Florida. More than 5,000 marathoners finish it each year. In addition to the marathon, the event also has a children's run the day before, a corporate relay, and a half marathon. To register, write Walt Disney World Marathon, P.O. Box 10,000, Lake Buena Vista, FL 32830; or call (407) 939-7810.

Disney Magic

The Walt Disney World Marathon is on my list because it's emblematic of an important trend in races, namely, making them family-friendly. We running geeks used to go pound the pavement while our families were left to kill the time until we crossed the finish line. But race organizers have discovered that it's better to involve as many members of the family as possible, rather than catering only to the hard-core marathoners.

Training Tip
When you plan a family trip in conjunction with a race, save most of your sight-seeing for the day or two after the race. You don't want to use a lot of physical and mental energy walking around an unfamiliar city before the race.

This family-friendly trend has grown as the average runner has become older and, therefore, more likely to have kids. Many races do a good job of making their weekend full of events for fit people of all ages and levels of seriousness. As the father of two young daughters, I like this emphasis and have enjoyed participating in Disney's family 5K the day before the marathon. Of course, families have plenty of other things they can do during race weekend deep in the heart of Walt Disney World!

For kids of all ages, Walt Disney's course has a certain charm. I grew up watching *The Wonderful World of Disney* on Sunday nights, so I'm a sucker for this stuff. Apparently, a lot of other "mature" runners are, too, if the number of people who rave every year about running through Cinderella's Castle is any proof.

Any Thanksgiving Race

Racing on Thanksgiving Day? Aren't you supposed to spend the day watching TV and overeating? What's next, racing on New Year's Eve? Well, I've done that, too, which may have been taking things a bit far, but there's nothing strange about going to a race on the most American of holidays. After all, what better way to work up an appetite for dinner?

Just the Facts

I'm guessing that you can figure out when these are held. Where are they? Believe it or not, in most towns that have a strong running community. Races on Thanksgiving Day morning have become as much of a celebratory running tradition as Fourth of July races. Check the sources I told you about in Chapter 18 to find a Thanksgiving Day race in your area.

Why Give Thanks on the Run?

The first road race of my life was the Manchester Road Race, a 4.75-miler held every Thanksgiving Day morning on the streets of Manchester, Connecticut. Even when I first did it, in 1966, it was a tradition-laden New England event. I won the high school division in a time of 25:18. At the time, it was the longest race of my life. I don't remember much about the race except that it seemed like an awfully long way. But I liked the feeling of being competent over this distance, which was more than what I was used to racing in high school races.

Rules of the Road
Line up with others who are going to be running at your predicted pace. If you start too far up front in the pack, you force faster runners to weave around you. This is discourteous to them and can be dangerous to you. Also, if you start too far in the front, you'll probably be hooked into starting at too fast of a pace and will suffer more at the end of the race because of it.

More than 20 years later, I was able to set a master's course record in that race. I haven't run the Manchester race in a while, but I always try to run in some event on Thanksgiving Day. You should, too. Why? To me, running a race is the ideal way to give thanks for having a healthy body that's under your control. Thanksgiving Day races, like most holiday events, are celebratory affairs. You're out there with your family and friends, you have a lot of fun with bunches of other runners, and then you head home for a great dinner. Most Thanksgiving Day races give portions of their entry fees to food banks, or they encourage runners to bring cans of food to help the less fortunate.

My Jingle Bell Runs

The Jingle Bell Runs are not just mine anymore, even though the official name is Bill Rodgers Jingle Bell Run. They're not races in the traditional sense, which is why they're on my list.

Just the Facts

My brother, Charlie, and I hold a few of these in the Boston area every year on different dates in December. These races are low-key *fun runs* of a few miles that raise money for charities. The largest one, in downtown Boston, attracts more than 3,000 runners. For more information, call my store, Bill Rodgers Running Center, at (617) 723-5612.

Jinglin' All the Way for Charity

I started holding these runs from my running store more than 20 years ago. At first, they weren't fundraisers for charity, just low-key runs with a few friends around the Boston Common and other parts of the city. We'd even stop at the tree outside of the Prudential Center and sing Christmas carols. It was a nice way to end the year after being so serious about training and racing so much of the time.

Now, the runs are a lot more organized, but they've kept that low-key feel to them. And we've made them fundraisers for different disabled children's groups. I'm a former special ed teacher, so this aspect means the world to me. I like it when runners can make the connection between doing this great thing for themselves, running, and helping others. Now, most big cities have similar affairs, and I think it's great that more runners have the chance to participate in these noncompetitive events and simultaneously do something for others.

The Race for the Cure Series

For you rock fans out there, sorry, but this series has nothing to do with that gloomy British band, The Cure. What it has to do with is a heck of a lot more important—finding a cure for breast cancer.

Just the Facts

The Race for the Cure is the largest series of 5K runs in the United States. In 1997, the series was held in 77 cities throughout the country and included nearly half a million participants. The Susan G. Komen Breast Cancer Foundation organizes this series of runs; proceeds from the runs provide funding for local and national breast cancer research, education, screening, and treatment programs. For more information, call (800) 653-5355; or visit the Web site, http://www.komen.org.

A Cure for Sure

In case you haven't noticed by now, I like it when there's a connection between running and the rest of society. Apparently, a lot of others do, too, because The Race for the Cure Series gets bigger and bigger every year. Just one event in the series, the Washington, DC one, is the single largest 5K in the country. Vice President Gore and his wife, Tipper, regularly run it, in part because of their family's history of breast cancer. That link exists for me, too, because my mom has had breast cancer. Many participants in these events are running in honor or memory of a breast cancer patient. Some in the field are even breast cancer survivors.

I have an ulterior motive in naming this among my favorite races: because of the emotional connection, The Race for the Cure Series draws a lot of participants who aren't part of the regular road racing scene. They're there to do their part to help conquer breast cancer, not necessarily to set the world on fire with their running. But having gotten a taste of the special, positive atmosphere that accompanies all races, many Race for the Cure runners find that they like the racing aspect of the sport and consequently become more active in other types of races. Events such as The Race for the Cure are a good way for running to broaden its organized participation base.

The Chase Corporate Challenge Series

Like the Race for the Cure Series, the Chase Corporate Challenge Series does a great job of luring new runners into the sport. It exposes occasional fitness runners to the racing scene and thereby shows them how fun it can be.

Just the Facts

The Chase Corporate Challenge Series consists of runs in 16 cities in the United States, plus two overseas. The series culminates in a national final held on Park Avenue in New York City in October. In all, more than 175,000 runners take part in the series each year. Each race features team awards as well as individual recognition, such as first executive finisher. Each race is 3.5 miles long—a good challenging distance for the serious racers, but also a conquerable distance for the more casual runner. To find out whether there's a series event near you, write Chase Corporate Challenge Series, 140 East 45th Street, 16th Floor, New York, NY 100017; or call (212) 622-8515.

Track Talk
A *fun run* is an untimed, short, low-key run, usually organized for charitable purposes. The idea is to run at a relaxed pace while enjoying yourself. Many big races hold fun runs in conjunction with the serious, timed event as a way to involve the racers' children and spouses who aren't interested in competition.

Rules of the Road
If others are accompanying you to a race, plan where and when you'll meet after the finish. Don't count on being able to find your spouse or friends as you mill about the finish area, especially when there are more than a few hundred runners in the race. Choose a spot at least a few hundred yards from the finish area.

There's No "I" in "Team"

In addition to introducing casual runners to the fun of racing, the Chase Corporate Challenge Series benefits runners in other ways. As you probably know, balancing your running with your work life can be tough. Work-based programs such as the Chase Series encourage employers to see their employees as more than just employees. They help show what employees do in the rest of their lives, and how important those pursuits are to them, and how having a healthy, rewarding life outside of work adds to, rather than detracts from, performance on the job. As mentioned in Chapter 3, the fittest employees are the ones who take the least number of sick days.

Training Tip
In most big races, it can take a couple of minutes to cross the starting line. If you wear a stopwatch, start it when you cross the starting line, rather than when the gun fires to start the race. Doing this will give you your actual running time over the course.

The Chase Corporate Challenge Series emphasizes a team approach that's often missing in running. Now don't get me wrong—I'm about as strong an individualist as you'll ever meet, and I like how running forces you to rely solely on yourself. At the same time, I started my running as a member of my high school and college cross-country and track teams. When I started running again after college, I almost immediately joined a team of runners who had goals similar to mine. As I keep emphasizing, running is just so much easier when you do it with others. In a Corporate Challenge race, you might not run side by side with fellow employees. But knowing that your co-workers are out there on the same course at the same time doing their best is a great way to motivate yourself. I'd like to see more events that explore the teamwork aspect of running that's so often ignored.

The Avon Mini Marathon

The only thing I don't like about the Avon Mini Marathon is its name. This race is a 10K (6.2 miles)—why call it a mini marathon? A marathon is 26.2 miles long; other races are their own babies. I mean, 100-meter dashes aren't called "mini miles!"

Just the Facts

This race is on my list even though I've never run it. Blame my parents for that, I guess, because I'm not allowed to run it—it's a women's-only 10K through New York City's Central Park, held the first Saturday in June. The tough course is a hilly loop around the park's perimeter. Nonetheless, more than 7,000 women run it each year, including some of the fastest in the world. The course record is 31:00, which converts to 5:00 miles for 6.2 hilly miles. The New York Road Runners Club puts on the race. For information, write NYRRC, 9 East 89th Street, New York, NY 10128; or call (212) 860-4455.

Footnotes

Because of unfounded concern about female frailty, the first Olympic Marathon for women wasn't held until 1984. Joan Benoit of the United States won in 2:24:52—a time that would have won every men's Olympic Marathon until 1952.

Ladies Only, Please

Some people might tell you that this women's-only race practices reverse sexism. After all, think what a stink would be raised if you held a men's-only race, right? Look, guys, as I said at the beginning of this chapter, there are more than 10,000 road races held in the United States every year. I think you can find ample competitive opportunities.

More important, the Avon Mini Marathon, along with other women's-only races such as the 7,000-runner Tufts 10K in Boston, attracts many women runners who might not otherwise enter a race. As I said in Chapter 17, I think all runners should go to races once in a while, even if they're not going to run any faster than on a regular training run. The celebratory atmosphere of races adds an element of excitement that you can't find on your standard runs around the neighborhood. But some women are intimidated by races, mostly because (usually unfoundedly so) they're afraid of finishing last. At these huge all-women races, these women feel more relaxed and have a greater sense of camaraderie.

If women's-only races are what it takes to get women to participate, then I'm all in favor of them. I have two daughters, and I like the idea of them having as many opportunities to be fit as boys do. Most races still have a disproportionate percentage of men in the field, so anything that helps bring the numbers closer to parity is worth it. And because the Mini Marathon is held in the media capital of the world, it usually gets some kind of TV coverage. It's important for women runners occasionally to be the sole focus of the media's attention.

Training Tip

In big races that have a lot of spectators, you can get a boost from the crowd by wearing a top printed with your name or that of a college. The people watching the race will see your top and cheer specifically for you, rather than clapping and offering general encouragement.

The Least You Need to Know

➤ To run the Boston Marathon, you need to qualify by finishing a marathon under certain standards in the year before.

➤ The New York City Marathon was the first marathon to be run through the streets of a major city, a model that has now been copied the world over.

➤ Some races are non-competitive fun runs that raise money for a variety of charitable causes.

➤ Races such as the Chase Corporate Challenge Series are team events that are a nice alternative to the usual focus on individual results.

➤ Women's-only races encourage participation from many women runners who might not otherwise attend races.

Part 5
Running Through the Ages

By now, I hope that I've gotten across to you that running is a lifetime sport, even a way of life. Running isn't just for fast, thin 25-year-olds. Children run, teens run, old geezers in their 50s like me run, and great-grandparents run.

Most of what I've said in this book applies to all runners. But in this part, you'll find out what runners at the two extremes of the age scale should know. I'll explain what kind of running is right for children and whether it's safe for senior citizens to start running. (Can you guess what the answer is?) Finally, in this part you'll discover how your running changes over the years when you stick with it, as well as what to do to keep running the sport of your life.

Kidding Around: Running for Children

One time my co-author, Scott Douglas, came over to my house. My younger daughter was in the driveway when Scott pulled up and asked him, "Are you here to see my daddy?" "Yes," Scott said. "Tell him Frank Shorter is here to see him." Erika ran into the house and told me that Frank had arrived. This was news to me—I was expecting Scott, not an impromptu visit from an old rival who lives on the other side of the country! I dashed out to the driveway and saw only Scott and realized that toying with a gullible five-year-old was his idea of a joke.

The reason that Scott's lame little ploy worked was because Erika doesn't know Frank Shorter from Frank Perdue or Frankenstein. That's good. At her age, I want her to take part in as many activities as she enjoys, not become some hard-core pre-teen running geek. If she wants to get immersed in my world, there's plenty of time for that later.

Encouraging children to be active without going overboard is what this chapter is about. I'll explain how much and why children should run and what types of races I think are good for them. I also have a few words for the older children out there who may have joined their high school cross-country or track team.

Should Children Run?

Of course children should run! Running should be as much a part of children's lives as walking, skipping, playing tag, and so on. It should be a normal part of their play. For preteens, play can and should be the major source of physical activity. Some researchers have estimated that when kids are left to their own devices, they'll cover as much as six miles a day on foot. Obviously, they don't cover this distance all at once, and it's a lot different from when an adult goes out for a six-mile run or walk, but that's OK. At that age, most experts would agree, what you want is for your children to be active in a variety of activities that they enjoy.

Training Tip
Children running 10 or more miles per week need good running shoes as much as adults do. Because their bones, muscles, tendons, and ligaments are still developing, young runners do best in shoes with good cushioning that will absorb much of the impact shock.

Of course, many kids aren't active. The average American teenager watches 22 hours of TV a week. Keep that in mind as you ponder these scary statistics: Only one-third of children ages 6 to 17 meet minimum standards of cardio-vascular fitness. Of children between the ages of 5 and 8, 40 percent are obese, meaning that they weigh at least 20 percent more than they should. According to one survey of children in grades 4 to 12, 49 percent of boys and 62 percent of girls get nine hours or less of physical activity each week. When you consider that these estimates likely include a lot of time standing around on a ball field during gym classes, the figures seem even worse.

Now the question of whether children should run changes. Should children run in an organized way, for fitness, the way that adults do? That one's a bit trickier to answer.

Be a Running Role Model

You certainly shouldn't force children into running. Little League syndrome is as bad in running as it is in baseball. Children can sense when you're pushing them into an activity. They might not resist immediately, but eventually they will.

Having fun consistently ranks as the top reason that kids give for participating in sports. For preteens, fun almost always means the here and now. Most preteens haven't developed what psychologists call abstract thinking, the ability to set long-term goals and to see how doing something that might not feel good right now is worth it for the pay-off later. In a certain sense, isn't that what a lot of running is about? A big motivation for getting out for a run today is because you know that doing so will benefit you later—

you'll feel better the next day, or you'll be able to run faster in a race a month from now, or you're working toward a weight-loss goal, or you're making one of an ongoing series of contributions to fighting disease, and so on. When children don't come to running on their own terms, they're not going to like it because they don't yet have that sense of delayed gratification.

If a kid wants to run and can state why and seems to enjoy it, then I'm all for some low-level regular running. Children's attitudes toward running largely stem from what they notice about how the adults around them approach it. If you're always walking around the house before your runs moaning about what a horrible chore running is, then don't be surprised if your kids don't show much interest in it. But if your children see that running to you means getting outside and exploring and feeling good and being with your friends and having fun, they'll probably think otherwise. Running will seem like a form of play.

Rules of the Road
Young runners should follow the same safety rules as adults, as laid out in Chapter 4. Running with others is an especially good safety guideline to follow.

Keep It Enjoyable!

Even if your kids want to run for all the right reasons, I don't think that children under the age of 14 should look at their running as training. This advice doesn't mean that children under this age can't run as much as 20 miles a week. If they want to run that much, enjoy doing so, and don't get hurt, I think that's an acceptable upper limit of mileage for preteens. Three miles or 30 minutes are good measures of the farthest that young runners should go at a time.

But although kids may run as much as adults, running should remain a part of their play and one of many regular activities, not something that they plan and obsess about. Going for a run should be primarily about enjoying it on that day, not to build endurance so that they can try to run twice as far in a month. This book has emphasized that if you're going to make progress in your running, then you need to be consistent with it. Kids who run should ignore all of that. If they hit a spell where they don't feel like running for a month or two, don't force them to. If you do, you're sending the message that running is something that they have to do, not that they want to do.

The Fun of Family Fitness

My wife and I like to introduce our two daughters to as many activities as possible. Sure, running is one of them, and it's kind of hard for them not to notice that it seems as though Daddy is always heading out the door for a run. But we never tell them how running is the greatest sport, or how they're wasting their time when they're skating, dancing, boating, playing basketball or tennis, or doing any of the other activities that they've found that they enjoy.

Training Tip
A good way to introduce kids to running and to solve the child-care question during your running time is to run on a track while they play on the infield. After awhile, they'll probably be interested enough to want to try to join you for a lap or two.

Training Tip
When running with children, let them lead the way. Run half a step behind so that it doesn't seem that they're always working to keep up with you. If you make them follow you, running will seem to be more of a chore than a form of play.

What we want to do is get across the idea that fitness is a lifestyle. We want to show them that being active and healthy and feeling good while using your body on a regular basis should be the norm. Children are much more likely to develop good fitness habits for the rest of their lives if they see that fitness is important to you. That's a much better message to send than presenting fitness as an occasional intrusion that you have to tend to out of obligation.

In terms of running, this approach means that if your child expresses an interest in it, explore that interest together. Go for a run with your kid. Take him or her to your races, not so much to run, but to show the festive atmosphere that races have. Do what you can to expose your child to those elements of running that are going to have the most appeal to kids.

You might not think so, but one of the biggest appeals of running is going to be the chance to spend some quality time with you. Young kids, especially, will do almost anything to get adult attention. So if they want to run with you, indulge them. Running together can strengthen your relationship, because the child will see your runs as one-on-one, undivided attention time. Let these runs unfold on the child's terms. That might mean jumping through puddles, or stopping to look at animals, or heading home after just a few minutes. Let them set the pace and the course. Remember, it's supposed to be fun for them, which means feeling good right then.

The Right Races for Rug Rats

In the 1970s, a young runner named Wesley Paul ran faster than 3:00 for the marathon at age 9, the youngest that anyone had ever done so. This feat got him a lot of attention in the press, and one running magazine even speculated that he would grow up to break the world record. You don't hear about Wesley Paul these days, however. That's not surprising. For whatever reason, almost every child who is highly motivated to compete in races at a young age doesn't become a lifetime runner. Probably for the same reason that kids who are gymnastics dynamos aren't big on tumbling when they're 40 years old—the activity is associated with a lot of pressure, not fun, and we all have enough pressure in our adult lives as it is.

I'm not a big fan of age-group track meets for junior high and elementary school kids. There's just too much of a risk that the children are so serious at such a young age for the wrong reasons. Sure, some of the runners might be mature enough to be able to state why they're training hard toward meeting competitive goals, but I'd rather err on the side of caution. Kids who have the ability and interest to become top runners will have plenty of time to work on that goal later, when both their minds and bodies are more mature, and they can make fuller use of their potential.

The Boston Marathon doesn't allow anyone under the age of 18 to enter the race. I support this position. There's no real benefit to be had from runners younger than that doing marathons, and the risks of burnout and injury are too great, given how much you have to run to prepare for a marathon. Hey, it's hard enough for adults to articulate reasonably why they want to try to run such a crazy distance!

So what kinds of races are good for kids who want to participate? I'm all in favor of the low-key, mostly noncompetitive children's fun runs that more and more road races have added. Both of my daughters have run in these types of events. The important thing to look for in these runs is that they're short enough that you know your child will be able to finish and that they encourage participation, not competition.

If the race is too long, it's going to be a frustrating experience for the child. Why would he or she want to fail? My older daughter's first event like this was one kilometer, or just more than half a mile, long. Anything more than 5K is asking for trouble. The child may stick it out and finish, but it sure won't be fun.

Rules of the Road

Young runners need to be especially careful in extreme weather. Children's bodies don't create as much heat as adults' bodies do, so they're at greater risk for hypothermia in cold weather. Children's cooling systems are similarly underdeveloped— they don't sweat as easily as adults, so they get hotter quicker in the summer.

Footnotes

In 1996, the Junior Bloomsday, a two-mile children's fun run held in conjunction with the Lilac Bloomsday 12K in Spokane, Washington, was the 37th largest road race in the United States. More than 8,000 kids took part!

Kids are naturally competitive. Watch the start of these children's runs, and you'll see the term "youthful exuberance" defined. They just tear away from the starting line in a sprint! But to keep the events fun and worthwhile for all the young runners, children's races should give some kind of award to every finisher. At a young age, the top finishers are going to place first because they have more talent for running. Preparing for the event doesn't factor into winning as it does for adults, especially at short distances.

Acknowledging all of the participants, by giving them all identical finisher's medals, for example, gets across the idea that the most important victory is participating. This emphasis encourages the slower kids to keep coming back and to view running as a sport that's for everyone, not just the talented few. Kids see enough of the elitist view of sports as it is, with the overemphasis that school sports such as football and basketball receive.

Teen Angels: High School Runners

Once kids are in high school, it's OK for them to become more serious about competition. By this age, they'll be able to understand what training is and how sometimes you have to suffer in the present to have a better future. Racing might still be frustrating (it is for everyone at some point), but if they've freely chosen to compete, then a few bad experiences probably won't sour them on running for the rest of their lives.

Footnotes

In the 1996-1997 school year, outdoor track and field was the second most popular high school sport among girls, following only basketball. For boys, track was third, behind football and basketball.

Also, by this age, their bodies can handle the training better. Training for even the longest distances usually offered in high school (5K for cross-country, two miles for track) involves a lot of short, fast speed work, usually on the track. By high school age, more runners are going to be able to do this type of training without breaking down.

Footnotes

The two basic types of scholastic track meets are a *dual meet* and an *invitational*. Dual meets involve a few schools, with the team title going to the school that amasses the most points. These meets are usually held during the school week. Invitationals are bigger affairs, usually held on weekends, that draw schools from throughout a region. The focus in these meets is more on performance in specific events than on team titles. Some invitationals have qualifying times.

Most children who race the mile or two-mile in outdoor track are going to top out at about 30 miles a week. Anything more than that, and I'd get a little wary. Certainly, some teens can handle more running than that, especially if they started when they were younger. But even in high school, I think it's worth erring on the side of caution.

Footnotes

Only three American high school students have broken 4:00 for the mile, the last one being Marty Liquori way back in 1967. The national high school record for boys is 3:55.3, held by Jim Ryun. For girls, the record is 4:35.2, held by Polly Plumer.

Some coaches are going to encourage members of the team to run more. It's not unheard of for cross-country team members to run 70 or so miles a week. Whether that's a good idea is going to be a judgment call. If a high school runner is doing that kind of mileage and understands why, then it can be OK, so long as the runners on the team are progressing and enjoying themselves. But if most members of the team aren't progressing, then the coach is trying to use methods that might work with older, more developed runners on younger ones who aren't ready yet for that high of a level of training. Because most high school runners are new to the sport, they should see steady progress in bringing their times down. If they've plateaued, it usually means that they're doing too much.

I ran a few road races while in high school. Doing a few short ones a year is fine for high school runners, especially as a way to keep running interesting in the summer. But I'm not in favor of teen runners being serious road racers. They should concentrate on the shorter track races and work on developing their speed and good training habits. When they're out of school, they have the rest of their lives to plod around on the roads like the rest of us. Once you're out of school, it's tough to find good competitions at short races like the mile. So teen runners should take full advantage of the opportunity while they have it. If they choose to compete when they're older, they'll be that much more able to reach their potential at the longer races.

Rules of the Road
Young runners should learn from day one a fundamental bit of runner's etiquette—to shake hands with the runners who place just ahead and behind them immediately after the finish of a race. This action encourages good sportsmanship and reinforces the notion that everyone in a race competes against themselves and the conditions, as well as other runners.

The Least You Need to Know

➤ Running should be one of many forms of children's play.

➤ Children will learn to view running favorably if they see it presented as something that's fun.

➤ The best races for pre-high schoolers are short, noncompetitive events that reward all of the participants.

➤ Children under the age of 18 shouldn't run marathons.

➤ It's OK for children to become more serious about training and competition once they're in high school.

➤ High school runners should focus on short races such as the mile rather than longer road races.

Chapter 25

Late in the Race: Advice for Senior Runners

> **In This Chapter**
>
> ➤ Why age doesn't matter
>
> ➤ Getting started after age 50
>
> ➤ Precautions for older new runners
>
> ➤ Special nutritional advice for older runners

When I turned 50 in December 1997, people made a big deal about it. They thought it was incredible that I was still running at such an advanced age. Some people wanted to know when I was going to retire. Never, I hope. Our society has it all wrong about aging. Our bodies are meant to be used for our entire lives, not just when we're young.

But what if you didn't even use your body back then? What if you've been sedentary for a long time, but now want to start running? Is it for you? In this chapter, I'll tell you why you have nothing to fear from starting a running program, as well as give you some tips to make the transition from 50 and fat to 60 and sexy easier.

All Ages Welcome

It's never too late to get in shape. People who start running in their 70s will see the same kinds of gains that people in their 20s do. The principles that underlie why your aerobic capacity and strength increase when you start running have no idea how old you are.

That's not what older people have traditionally been told. People past the age of 60 were told to take it easy—maybe putter around the garden a couple of times a week or walk the dog (assuming the dog is no bigger than a dachshund). Get the old ticker going, and you'll be pushing up daisies, not pulling in Social Security. Getting sick and increasingly dependent on others is an inevitable part of getting old, we were told.

Now we know that that advice, like history, is bunk. As one of the leading researchers in this area likes to say, what most people think of as the natural consequences of aging are really the "atrophy of disuse." Our bodies are machines that like being used. Start them up at a good rate after years of practicing "atrophy of disuse," and they will thank you for it.

One study started a group of sedentary men in their 60s on a walking and running program. They worked out four times a week for 30 minutes at 70 percent of their maximum heart rate. (Sound familiar? See Chapter 3.) After only four weeks, their aerobic capacity had increased by six percent, and their heart rate at their training pace decreased by 10 beats per minute. After another five weeks, they had another six percent increase in aerobic capacity, and their training heart rate fell another six beats.

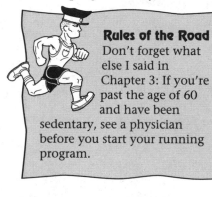

Rules of the Road
Don't forget what else I said in Chapter 3: If you're past the age of 60 and have been sedentary, see a physician before you start your running program.

Training Tip
Older runners can especially benefit from weight training. In general, older runners tend to get ankle and knee injuries and tendinitis around the joints. Weight training helps to protect joints by strengthening the tissues around them, which results in fewer injuries.

Older people can benefit from strength training as well. One of the main reasons that older people lose independence, and with it, quality of life, is because they've lost so much muscle mass that they can't perform basic daily tasks. Being unable to lift more than five pounds might not seem like much of a big deal until you do some quick math: Half a gallon of milk weighs three pounds. Go to the store and buy that, a few pieces of fruit, and maybe some chicken breast, and you better be able to lift more than five pounds unless you want to rely on others to carry even the lightest groceries for you.

A famous study at Tufts University started frail people in their 80s on a serious weight training program. The old folks did repetitions at 80 percent of their one-rep maximum. That's hard work for anyone, believe me. In just eight weeks, their strength more than doubled.

The bottom line: Not only can older sedentary people start an exercise program like younger people, but they should. The benefits of exercise, as well as the principles for obtaining these benefits, are the same no matter what your age.

278

Leaving Youth in the Dust

If you're over the age of 50 and have been sedentary for a long time, do you remember how you felt more than 20 years ago? Probably pretty darned good, huh? Even if you weren't brimming with vitality, you probably wouldn't mind feeling like that again instead of how you feel now, right? Well, if you start running, you can feel that way again.

A study of runners age 50 and older compared them to healthy nonrunners in their 20s. The women runners had an average level of aerobic fitness the same as the sedentary 20-somethings, and the 50+ men runners had slightly higher aerobic capacities than the young couch potatoes. Based on these figures, you could say that running cuts 20 to 30 years from your age!

Footnotes

Think we oldtimers can't duke it out with the young bucks? John Campbell placed fourth at the 1990 Boston Marathon at age 41. His time of 2:11:04 is a world record for a masters runner. The man whose record he broke, Jack Foster, ran a 2:20 marathon at age 50.

Retired Runners

People today switch not just jobs, but careers several times in their work years. That wasn't usually the case for the generation of people now retiring. These were the company men—you got a job with Industrial Behemoth, Inc. when you were young, and you stayed there until you retired. You weren't encouraged to do much more than be an employee, a husband, and a father. The women were encouraged to stay home and raise the kids while tending to the endless household chores. You didn't have hobbies; you had responsibilities.

But what now? You've retired, the kids are long gone and that dream of hours of leisure time might have become a nightmare. Throughout this book, I've shown how running is not just exercise; it's a lifestyle. No, you're not going to spend your entire day running, but it does help to center your day. Having this activity on your schedule has a way of organizing your day; there seems to be more of a purpose to what you do. I keep mentioning how running improves the quality of your life. This benefit is especially important for older people, who suffer from depression at a higher rate than young people.

Footnotes

Late in his 60s, Maryland's Ed Benham began running at the urging of his sons. They thought it would help Ed deal with being a widower. Benham went on to set innumerable records for men of his age. In 1989, at age 81, he ran 1:13:23 for 10 miles, which is faster than 7:30 per mile!

One of the most amazing runners I know of is Warren Utes of Park Forest, Illinois. Utes began running in 1978 at age 58. When he retired in 1985, he had several years of base behind him and went on a running rampage that hasn't stopped. Among his many records are a 39:41 10K at age 74, making him the oldest person ever to break 40:00 for the distance. Need me to do the math? That's almost 6:20 per mile for 6.2 miles! Utes runs 60 miles a week and is having the time of his life. Wouldn't you like to join him?

Masterful Performances

OK, so you're pretty fired up about all that running has to offer older people. Is there anything special you need to do besides rereading the chapters in the first section of this book? Yes, there is. Although the principles for getting fit are the same for everybody, they do require a slightly different application in an older body. How much is going to be different depends on how active you are. If the last time you got any exercise was when you hoisted beers in college, you're going to have to start much more slowly than if you've always walked places, played tennis once in a while, chased after the grandchildren, and so on.

What doesn't differ is the fact that all people should start their exercise programs with that basic 30 minutes, four-times-a-week approach where you work hard enough to work up a sweat, but not so hard that you can't carry on a conversation. At what level of activity this occurs depends on how well you've taken care of yourself. Be honest about what it takes at first to reach the right workout intensity. Don't let visions of your former self cloud your perception of your current reality.

Rules of the Road
Be mindful of old injuries from other sports. That knee that you wrenched playing football years ago might become a lot more noticeable when you start to run. See a good sports medicine doctor if you have an old injury site that bothers you when you start running.

Some people in their 60s are able to start running right away, but a lot of older people have to walk at first. Whether you start off running or walking, you're getting the aerobic benefits of exercise, and you're building good workout habits. We older folks don't need instant gratification as much as the youngsters. We're used to working at something that has a promise of future reward. I hope by now that I've convinced you what a great reward is waiting for you if you stick with your running.

Slow and Steady

As I'll talk about in more length in the next chapter, one of the biggest changes that happens to your body as you age is that your ability to recover from a hard workout decreases. Most older runners find that they need to allow for extra time between hard workouts, or they'll risk injury. For long-time runners, making this adjustment is one of the trickiest aspects of getting older. When you were in your 30s, you had no trouble putting in long hours at the office, cranking out a good speed workout in the middle of the week, and racing or doing a long run on the weekend. So you wonder why doing so now takes so much out of you.

One of the beauties of beginning to run when you're older is that you don't have those memories. You don't have to worry about how to adjust the running schedule that used to work for you. But you still should be aware that all other things being equal, you're not going to recover from your workouts as quickly as new runners in their 20s. If they go overboard at first and get a lot sorer than they should, it's not that big a deal. They'll be fine in a couple of days. You on the other hand…

Be extra careful about running within your limits at first. Finish each of your workouts feeling that you could have kept going or that you could have done the workout at a faster clip. Try to maintain that little bit of extra conservatism for at least the first six months of your running program.

Be Flexible

Older beginners should also be extra diligent about a good flexibility program. Young new runners are limited mostly by their aerobic fitness. If they can't go faster, it's because their muscles, heart, and lungs need to develop the capacity to sustain a higher level of effort. But if they had to, they could launch into a full sprint and look pretty good doing it.

But older runners, especially ones who have been sedentary, have another limitation. They've probably lost a good deal of their range of motion over the years. If they tried to break into a sprint, they might very well trip over their feet or at least risk pulling something.

Training Tip
A lot of how you adapt to running has to do with your attitude. "The word 'training' is obnoxious to me," says New Zealand's Derek Turnbull. "When I run, it's for recreation. Fitness is half in the mind—if you enjoy your running, you'll get results." This is from a man who ran a 2:47 marathon in his mid 60s!

Rules of the Road
If you used to work out, but haven't in more than a few years, you're starting from scratch. Don't try to match what you used to do, especially if you're comparing your current self to when you were in your 20s and 30s.

Running will help you to regain some of your range of motion as your muscles become used to working harder. But you can help them to help you by stretching regularly. For younger beginners, stretching is mostly going to maintain flexibility. But for older runners, stretching can improve your flexibility, helping you to regain some of that agility that you used to take for granted. This improvement can be exciting for older folks who have gotten used to not moving as well as they used to.

Aging Appetites

The basic nutritional lowdown that I gave you in Chapter 13 applies to all runners. No matter what your age, you should eat a low-fat, high-carbohydrate diet to get the most out of your running. That said, older runners can benefit from tweaking their diet a bit.

As always, the most important advice has to do with fluids, not food. Everyone's thirst mechanisms are pretty lame at keeping them well-hydrated. But as you age, your thirst mechanism becomes even less sensitive. To make matters worse, runners past the age of 40 have higher core body temperatures, heart rates, and overall loss of body water in the heat than younger runners do. It's a double whammy—if you're not careful, you start a run in the heat less hydrated, then have the heat take more out of you. So older runners should be even more zealous about staying hydrated than younger ones. Remember to drink some fluid every hour that you're awake, and check that your urine is frequent and clear in color.

Footnotes

The oldest person ever to break 3:00 for the marathon is John Keston of McMinnville, Oregon. Six months before his 70th birthday, he ran 2:58:33, placing eighth out of 208 runners. Keston holds the world record for 70-and-older runners with a 3:00:58 marathon.

Your stomach produces less acid as you age, which reduces your ability to digest protein. Most people find that a big steak just isn't as appealing when they're 60 as it was when they were 20. Overall, that's good, because, as I mentioned in Chapter 13, most people eat too much protein as it is. Still, older runners who don't have much of an appetite for animal products should make sure that they're getting their two to three servings of protein a day, or recovering from illness or injury is going to take longer.

Older women runners should be sure to get enough calcium. Yes, running helps to keep bones strong, but after menopause, estrogen levels plummet, and bones can become more brittle if you don't take in enough calcium. When this happens, you're more susceptible to stress fractures from your running.

Aging decreases your skin's ability to produce vitamin D. Many older runners, myself included, are rightfully concerned about skin cancer and wear sunscreen. Also, older runners are more likely to find themselves running at nonpeak sun hours because of work and family responsibilities. All of this means that masters runners should take extra steps to get enough vitamin D through their diet, which works with calcium to keep your bones strong. Fortified nonfat milk is the best source.

The good news is that older runners get to eat more calories than their sedentary contemporaries. This means that it's more possible to eat enough of a variety of foods to take in the nutrients you need.

The Least You Need to Know

➤ New runners past the age of 50 get the same benefits from running as younger runners do.

➤ Older beginning runners should work out just as hard as younger beginners.

➤ Older runners should stretch diligently to regain range of motion.

➤ Older runners have a decreased thirst sensation and need to be extra careful about drinking enough water.

Running for Your Life

In This Chapter

➤ Running even when you become slower

➤ Maintaining strength and flexibility as you age

➤ Staying motivated as the years go by

➤ The greatest athlete in American history

I started running when John F. Kennedy was president. After dabbling in a summer track meet put on by the local recreation department, me, my brother Charlie, and my best friend, Jason Kehoe, went out for the high school cross-country team. We found out how much fun running is, so we didn't quit the team. Now, 35 years later, you know what? We're all still running. We keep discovering new ways that running is fun. I don't think that any of us will be quitting the team anytime soon.

Running is a lifetime sport. In this chapter, I'll show you what changes happen over the years if you keep at it, and I'll show you how to make aging a positive thing, not a cause for despair. I'll conclude this book by telling you who the greatest athlete in American history is.

Do Not Go Gentle into That Good Night

What the Irish poet Dylan Thomas wrote to his aging father is good advice for all of us: Rage, rage against the dying of the light.

Our notions of what getting older is supposed to be about are wrong. They're based more on observing what people do, not what they should do. Use it or lose it is certainly true concerning fitness in the short term. As we've seen, your aerobic capacity starts to decline after as little as two weeks of inactivity.

If that's the case, think about what happens over the years. People who say they want to "take it easy" now that they're getting older have a self-fulfilling goal. Take it easy, and trust me, that's all you'll be capable of.

Think about the more interesting older people whom you've met in your life. What did they have in common? They were active. Sure, they probably weren't out there banging out the miles every day, but they did *something*. They had something in their lives that they were passionate about, that they applied their mental and physical abilities toward. That's why they remained interesting people—they had found some pursuit that they enjoyed, that gave meaning and order to their lives.

It's not so much that they rebelled against our society's encouragement of giving in to inertia, but that they ignored it. They just went about their business, and happened to get older along the way. Haven't you ever noticed how so many classical music conductors are still leading orchestras at ages when most people have gone deaf to doing anything but sitting in a rocking chair?

You don't have to be a world-class musician to live this way, and you don't have to be a former world-class runner, like me. You just need to find something that you care about, then keep pursuing it, open to where it might take you. Do that, and incidentally, you'll stay physically and mentally sharp enough to rage against the dying of the light.

Don't know if you saw this coming, but if not, here it is: Running is one of the best ways to live the rest of your life like this.

Through the Years: How Aging Affects Running

Going bald is a good analogy for what's going to happen to you if you keep running as you age. The changes are subtle, almost imperceptible from day to day. You can't point to one day and say, "That's when it all started." But a look in the mirror or the training log reveals that you're undeniably different. What you used to take for granted is now the stuff of fantasy.

If you're a performance-driven runner (and aren't we all to some degree?), you'll eventually find out the biggest change that happens to you when you get older: You slow down. You probably knew that already, but what you may not know is why that occurs and what you can do about it.

Recovering Performance Addicts

One of the first-noticed and universal changes that runners note with age is a decreased ability to recover after a long or hard run. When Frank Shorter was at his peak, he would do his longest run of the week on Sunday morning and be recovered enough by Monday afternoon to do speed work on the track. If he tried that now, it would kill him or at least kill any hope he would have of being able to walk for a week.

I've had to accept this change in my running as well. When I was training to be the best in the world, I cranked out 130-mile weeks with relative ease. (Don't let anyone tell you it's ever completely easy!) Now, I peak at about 90 miles a week, with 70 a more typical weekly mileage figure. But I'm more tired now doing that than I was when I used to do twice as much.

Mileage aside, I just feel, well, older. I still have the energy to do the things that I want to do, but I'm more aware of being tired when doing them. When I get up in the morning, it takes me awhile to get going. On days when I'm not pressed for time, I sometimes putter around the house for more than an hour before heading out for my run. I used to be able to start a run immediately, anytime, anywhere. Now, I need to walk around a bit, loosen up, and make a more conscious effort to get myself out the door.

Most long-time runners find that they need to allow for more easy days in their training and that they need to put more easy days between their hard workouts. Instead of running five miles the day after a track workout, maybe they'll do some cross-training or not do any exercise. That way, they'll recover better in time for that long run in a few days.

Another approach is to scrap the idea of looking at your training in week-long blocks. Instead of thinking that you have to get in a long run and a speed workout session every week and tweaking your easy days in whatever way is necessary to make that schedule fit, you could think in 10-day blocks, or 12-day ones, or whatever. You might just run easy after a hard workout until you feel ready to go hard again and not care whether that means three days or four or two.

Footnotes

A study comparing 50-and-over runners with runners in their 20s found that the older runners had better training routines, such as regularly stretching, than the younger ones. Appreciate aging for how it motivates you and rewards you for good habits.

There's a positive aspect about this reduced ability to recover from run to run. You become more conscious of the need to take care of yourself. You become better at finessing things in such a way to keep you on the roads. You probably acquire better habits, such as being diligent about stretching and maintaining a proper diet, because you have a better sense of how these things contribute to feeling better.

VO₂ Min?

Studies have found that after the age of 30, aerobic capacity drops by one percent each year. This means that everything else being equal, you're going to get a little slower each year. But not enough research has been done to distinguish how much of the decline that's observed in long-time runners is because of age and how much is due to training and living differently. My aerobic capacity is lower than it was 20 years ago. Some of that is inevitable, but how much of it is because I don't run as much as I used to? If my body would hold together at 130 miles per week, I bet my decline wouldn't be as great.

Footnotes

Aerobic fitness drops more because of inactivity than because of aging. In 1968, Lou Castagnola was a 2:17 marathoner. After the Olympic Marathon Trials that year, he stopped running completely. When he was retested just three years later, his aerobic capacity had decreased by more than 30 percent!

Aerobic capacity declines at a slower rate if you keep running. If you're running 20 miles a week now, that's a level that you will probably be to handle 10 years from now. You can therefore duplicate the standards of your heyday a lot more easily than I can. Your drop isn't going to be as great as mine.

Remember, your aerobic capacity improves for the first several years of a running program. If you're starting out as a runner after the age of 30, your aerobic capacity is going to increase from your training a lot more than it will decrease because of aging. As explained in the last chapter, that can mean that runners in their 50s have the capabilities of average people in their 20s. Just remember that the more aerobic exercise you get, the longer your aerobic capacity will take to decline.

Fast Twitchin'

When you run fast, you're using your *fast-twitch muscle fibers*. Everyone is born with a set percentage of fast-twitch fibers. If you have a lot of them, you'll be better at short races. If you weren't born with many (as I wasn't), then you have a higher percentage of slow-twitch fibers, the types that don't fire as quickly, but that can keep firing for a long time. If that's you, you'll be better at longer events. Differences in the percentages of fast-twitch and slow-twitch muscle fibers go a long way toward explaining why Carl Lewis is never going to run a good marathon and why I'm not a sprinter.

All muscle fibers degenerate with age, but fast-twitch fibers do so the quickest. Research indicates that if fast-twitch fibers aren't used regularly with age, their ability to fire is lost permanently. They kind of go into early retirement, and no amount of coaxing is going to bring them back. When this happens, you're going to lose your ability to move quickly, not just when running, but when doing daily activities.

You can't increase the percentage of your fast-twitch fibers with training, but you can increase their ability to work hard. You do this by doing things that require them to fire, such as doing striders and lifting weights regularly.

> **Track Talk**
> *Fast-twitch fibers* are muscle fibers that fire quickly to power explosive activities, such as sprinting or lifting weights. You're born with a set percentage of fast-twitch fibers, but you can keep the ones that you have activated by including fast running and strength training in your fitness program.

Lift for Life

Related to the degeneration of fast-twitch fibers is the loss of muscle mass. This loss means that you lose strength, and that you're more likely to gain weight. The old saw about muscle turning into fat isn't true—biochemically speaking, they're different materials—but it sure can seem that way. What happens is that when you lose some muscle mass, your metabolism slows. When that happens, it's easier to eat more calories than you burn, so it's easier for your body to gain fat.

But as explained in the last chapter, people of any age can increase their strength and add muscle with weight training. One of the best things you can do to keep your running rewarding as you age is to become more diligent about lifting weights.

It's Not a Stretch to Say...

Some decline in flexibility is inevitable. Muscles lose their resiliency over time. But most of why people are less flexible with age is because of their habits. As many runners age, they increasingly avoid running fast. Doing so feels tougher than it used to, so they stick with their easy daily runs. But this slower pace means that they're not working through a full range of motion like they should be. They're shuffling down the street, thinking about how much more difficult it is these days to run fast. But part of that is because they're shuffling down the street!

To combat this decline, do striders once or twice a week, even if you're not going to race. Striders are short enough that they're not going to tire you, but they require enough change in your running form that you're going to stretch your running muscles more than if you always run at just a moderate pace.

For many people, getting older means more days spent sitting behind a desk. Sitting all day shortens your hamstrings, tightens your lower back, and places tremendous strain on your neck. It detracts from your ability to move smoothly, especially in something like running where all of your body parts work in sync. A little regular stretching goes a long way toward keeping you from getting too creaky. Keep in mind that as you age, you have to keep doing your stretching routine just to maintain your flexibility.

Coping Strategies

When you're new to running, staying motivated is often easier than when you've been running for a while. If you follow some of the strategies in Chapter 6, you'll find ways to keep at it past your initial gains in fitness. Racing, especially, will help you to stay on track, so to speak, because you're likely to be fired up about chasing new personal records.

But what about when you realize that there won't be any more personal records? Isn't running just going to depress you? Well, it's been 15 years since the last time I set a personal record, and in some ways, I'm enjoying my running more than ever. It's not that I don't care about my running times any more. I do, fanatically. But I've broadened my appreciation of running.

Training Tip
When your times get slower, keep things in perspective. They might still be better than you think. When I was 49, I ran 52:22 for 10 miles. That's 5:14 per mile. When I was 15 years old, I ran a one-mile race in 5:20. Three and a half decades later, I was a better runner than when I was in my teens!

There's more to continuing to enjoy your running as you get older than doing striders and lifting weights. Much of your satisfaction (and therefore, motivation) is going to come from the right mental approach. Now that I'm past 50, I have a better sense of how running improves my life in ways that I pretty much used to take for granted. The health and fitness benefits of running have become more important to me. I realize now that if for some reason I was told I could never race again, I'd still run for an hour a day. I didn't think that way when I was younger. When I finished college, I wasn't motivated to race any more, so I stopped running entirely. I didn't have that sense of how running improves all of the areas of my life that I do now.

As I said, I'm still pretty darned fired up about racing. One good way to stay motivated is to shift gears and take on different goals. For example, I haven't raced a marathon in more than five years now. I stopped doing so because getting to the starting line in good enough shape to perform as I wanted was too taxing. The training that I wanted to do to race a good marathon was too much, and I kept breaking down. I realized that I would need to focus on other distances if I was going to keep at it.

This change has been good for me. All runners should become a different type of runner at different times in their running lives. I run a lot more 5Ks than I used to. Not being a fast-twitch kind of guy, this isn't my area of expertise, but I like the challenge. It emphasizes a slightly different way to train, and that variety helps to keep me interested. Many runners find that they have an increased appreciation for short races as they age. Some even turn to track meets and race distances of a mile or shorter. It's satisfying to give that brief, all-out effort and know that the race is short enough that it's not going to drain you for days.

At the other extreme, many post-personal record runners turn to increasingly longer distances. *Ultramarathons*, or are drawing bigger fields every year. People who have run marathons like the challenge of seeing whether they can extend their distance. Ultramarathons are so long that you can't run them faster than your usual training pace, so there's not that pressure to count every second. Many people find that they recover from ultramarathons more quickly than from marathons because you have to run them at so relaxed a pace. Older runners do exceptionally well in ultramarathons, because maturity is really rewarded in these how-long-can-you-last affairs.

I'm not saying that everyone should go out and sign up for the next 50-miler. I've never run an ultramarathon, and I doubt I ever will. But you can get a lot of satisfaction out of testing the limits of your endurance. That might mean moving up from 5Ks to 10Ks or seeing whether you can work up to running 10 miles at a time if the longest run of your life is 5 miles.

Track Talk
Races that are longer than marathons are *ultramarathons*. The most common distance for ultramarathons is 50 miles.

As I mentioned in Chapter 17 when I told you about masters racing, another good way to keep a fresh outlook is to wipe the slate clean every five years. By comparing your efforts to those of your recent past, you can maintain that sense of excitement about your running. Changing your goals like this isn't giving in. You're in control of the process; it's just that you have to take different factors into consideration.

Finally, it helps to keep things in perspective. Not being able to run as fast as you used to might not be cause for elation, but it's not the apocalypse either. I hope by now you see that running has so much to offer that, like me, it's the thought of not doing it all, rather than doing it more slowly than you used to, that's the legitimate fear. Older runners sometimes point out that their running is the same as it used to be. They're still out there running for 30 minutes to an hour. They're covering less ground than they used to in that time, but that doesn't change the fundamental experience of their daily run.

The Greatest Athlete in American History

The greatest American athlete ever is Johnny Kelley. After he dropped out of the 1956 Boston Marathon, he thought that maybe it was time that he retired from running. Sure, he had won the race twice, in 1935 and 1945, and he had placed second seven times. But the last time that had happened was ten years ago, in 1946. Since then, he had fallen farther and farther behind the leaders. Now, he had dropped out. He was 47 years old. He obviously wasn't going to win again. Why not just give up the whole thing and lead a normal life?

Kelley decided to stick with it, and he finished 13th at Boston the next year. The next year, he finished Boston again. And he kept finishing it, year after year. Kelley finished the Boston Marathon for the last time in 1991, when at age 83, he ran 5:42. It was the 58th time he had completed the race.

Footnotes

Clarence DeMar won the Boston Marathon seven times, more than anybody else. He was 42 at the time of his last victory. When he was 50, he placed seventh. Even in 1954, at the age of 65, he placed 78th in a field of 153 runners.

Kelley is my hero. He's pure inspiration, a model for how we're supposed to live. He shows us that being an athlete isn't just being a young guy who gets paid millions of dollars to throw a football or hit a baseball for 5 or 10 years, and then let themselves go to pot. Athletes keep at their sport their whole lives, always pursuing their passion, always striving to get the best out of themselves. Being an athlete isn't something that gets in the way of your life; it's something that gives meaning to your life. Kelley exemplifies this idea.

This notion is still foreign in the United States, but people from other countries sometimes appreciate it. After he won the Boston Marathon for the third consecutive time in 1995, Kenyan Cosmas Ndeti was asked if he would be back for next year's race. Ndeti said, "I want to be like Johnny Kelley. I want to win 100 times."

I, too, want to be like Johnny Kelley. Now 90, he still runs every day, rising early to run along the ocean near his home in Cape Cod. I hope that this book has convinced you that that's a good goal for you. And I hope you see by now that it's a reachable one. Let's always run!

The Least You Need to Know

➤ Eventually, you're going to get slower as you age.

➤ Most of why people get slower is because of how they train not just because they're getting older.

➤ Running striders and lifting weights regularly will help you to maintain your strength and range of motion.

➤ Getting older often means coming to appreciate your running more.

➤ Johnny Kelley, who finished the Boston Marathon 58 times, is the greatest athlete in American history.

Runner's Pace Chart

Pace per mile	1 mile	2 miles	3 miles	5K (3.1 miles)	4 miles	5 miles	6 miles	10K (6.2 miles)
6:00	6:00	12:00	18:00	18:39	24:00	30:00	36:00	37:18
6:10	6:10	12:20	18:30	19:10	24:40	30:50	37:00	38:20
6:20	6:20	12:40	19:00	19:41	25:20	31:40	38:00	39:22
6:30	6:30	13:00	19:30	20:12	26:00	32:30	39:00	40:24
6:40	6:40	13:20	20:00	20:43	26:40	33:20	40:00	41:26
6:50	6:50	13:40	20:30	21:14	27:20	34:10	41:00	42:28
7:00	7:00	14:00	21:00	21:45	28:00	35:00	42:00	43:30
7:10	7:10	14:20	21:30	22:16	28:40	35:50	43:00	44:32
7:20	7:20	14:40	22:00	22:47	29:20	36:40	44:00	45:34
7:30	7:30	15:00	22:30	23:18	30:00	37:30	45:00	46:36
7:40	7:40	15:20	23:00	23:49	30:40	38:20	46:00	47:38
7:50	7:50	15:40	23:30	24:20	31:20	39:10	47:00	48:40
8:00	8:00	16:00	24:00	24:51	32:00	40:00	48:00	49:42
8:10	8:10	16:20	24:30	25:22	32:40	40:50	49:00	50:44
8:20	8:20	16:40	25:00	25:53	33:20	41:40	50:00	51:46
8:30	8:30	17:00	25:30	26:24	34:00	42:30	51:00	52:48
8:40	8:40	17:20	26:00	26:55	34:40	43:20	52:00	53:50
8:50	8:50	17:40	26:30	27:26	35:20	44:10	53:00	54:52
9:00	9:00	18:00	27:00	27:57	36:00	45:00	54:00	55:54
9:10	9:10	18:20	27:30	28:28	36:40	45:50	55:00	56:56
9:20	9:20	18:40	28:00	28:59	37:20	46:40	56:00	57:58
9:30	9:30	19:00	28:30	29:30	38:00	47:30	57:00	59:00
9:40	9:40	19:20	29:00	30:01	38:40	48:20	58:00	1:00:02
9:50	9:50	19:40	29:30	30:32	39:20	49:10	59:00	1:01:04
10:00	10:00	20:00	30:00	31:03	40:00	50:00	1:00:00	1:02:06
10:10	10:10	20:20	30:30	31:34	40:40	50:50	1:01:00	1:03:08
10:20	10:20	20:40	31:00	32:05	41:20	51:40	1:02:00	1:04:10
10:30	10:30	21:00	31:30	32:36	42:00	52:30	1:03:00	1:05:12
10:40	10:40	21:20	32:00	33:07	42:40	53:20	1:04:00	1:06:14
10:50	10:50	21:40	32:30	33:38	43:20	54:10	1:05:00	1:07:16

continues

continued

Pace per mile	1 mile	2 miles	3 miles	5K (3.1 miles)	4 miles	5 miles	6 miles	10K (6.2 miles)
11:00	11:00	22:00	33:00	34:09	44:00	55:00	1:06:00	1:08:18
11:10	11:10	22:20	33:30	34:40	44:40	55:50	1:07:00	1:09:20
11:20	11:20	22:40	34:00	35:11	45:20	56:40	1:08:00	1:10:22
11:30	11:30	23:00	34:30	35:42	46:00	57:30	1:09:00	1:11:24
11:40	11:40	23:20	35:00	36:13	46:40	58:20	1:10:00	1:12:26
11:50	11:50	23:40	35:30	36:44	47:20	59:10	1:11:00	1:13:28
12:00	12:00	24:00	36:00	37:15	48:00	1:00:00	1:12:00	1:15:30

Pace per mile	10 miles	Half-marathon (13.1 miles)	15 miles
6:00	1:00:00	1:18:39	1:30:00
6:10	1:01:40	1:20:50	1:32:30
6:20	1:03:20	1:23:01	1:35:00
6:30	1:05:00	1:25:13	1:37:30
6:40	1:06:40	1:27:23	1:40:00
6:50	1:08:20	1:29:34	1:42:30
7:00	1:10:00	1:31:32	1:45:00
7:10	1:11:40	1:33:57	1:47:30
7:20	1:13:20	1:36:08	1:50:00
7:30	1:15:00	1:38:20	1:52:30
7:40	1:16:40	1:40:30	1:55:00
7:50	1:18:20	1:42:42	1:57:30
8:00	1:20:00	1:44:52	2:00:00
8:10	1:21:40	1:47:02	2:02:30
8:20	1:23:20	1:49:15	2:05:00
8:30	1:25:00	1:51:25	2:07:30
8:40	1:26:40	1:53:07	2:10:00
8:50	1:28:20	1:55:18	2:12:30
9:00	1:30:00	1:58:00	2:15:00
9:10	1:31:40	2:00:11	2:17:30
9:20	1:33:20	2:02:22	2:20:00
9:30	1:35:00	2:04:33	2:22:30
9:40	1:36:40	2:06:44	2:25:00
9:50	1:38:20	2:08:55	2:27:30
10:00	1:40:00	2:11:07	2:30:00
10:10	1:41:40	2:13:17	2:32:30

Pace per mile	10 miles	Half-marathon (13.1 miles)	15 miles
10:20	1:43:20	2:15:28	2:35:00
10:30	1:45:00	2:17:40	2:37:30
10:40	1:46:40	2:19:50	2:40:00
10:50	1:48:20	2:22:01	2:42:30
11:00	1:50:00	2:24:12	2:45:00
11:10	1:51:40	2:26:23	2:47:30
11:20	1:53:20	2:28:34	2:50:00
11:30	1:55:00	2:30:45	2:52:30
11:40	1:56:40	2:32:56	2:55:00
11:50	1:58:20	2:35:08	2:57:30
12:00	2:00:00	2:37:19	3:00:00

Pace per mile	20 miles	Marathon (26.2 miles)
6:00	2:00:00	2:37:19
6:10	2:03:20	2:41:41
6:20	2:06:40	2:46:03
6:30	2:10:00	2:50:25
6:40	2:13:20	2:54:47
6:50	2:16:40	2:59:09
7:00	2:20:00	3:03:03
7:10	2:23:20	3:07:55
7:20	2:26:40	3:12:17
7:30	2:30:00	3:16:39
7:40	2:33:20	3:21:01
7:50	2:36:40	3:25:23
8:00	2:40:00	3:29:45
8:10	2:43:20	3:34:07
8:20	2:46:40	3:38:29
8:30	2:50:00	3:42:51
8:40	2:53:20	3:47:13
8:50	2:56:40	3:51:35
9:00	3:00:00	3:56:00
9:10	3:03:20	4:00:19
9:20	3:06:40	4:04:41
9:30	3:10:00	4:09:03
9:40	3:13:20	4:13:25

continues

continued

Pace per mile	20 miles	Marathon (26.2 miles)
9:50	3:16:40	4:17:50
10:00	3:20:00	4:22:12
10:10	3:23:20	4:26:34
10:20	3:26:40	4:30:56
10:30	3:30:00	4:35:19
10:40	3:33:20	4:39:40
10:50	3:36:40	4:44:02
11:00	3:40:00	4:48:24
11:10	3:43:20	4:52:46
11:20	3:46:40	4:57:08
11:30	3:50:00	5:01:30
11:40	3:53:20	5:05:52
11:50	3:56:40	5:10:15
12:00	4:00:00	5:14:38

Resources for Runners

Organizations

American College of Sports Medicine

P.O. Box 144

Indianapolis, IN 46206

Phone: (317) 637-9200

The members of this professional organization are primarily sports medicine and exercise science professionals. This organization regularly disseminates information to the public on the latest in exercise science and nutrition based on the research of its members. It also publishes *Medicine & Science in Sports & Exercise*, a monthly, peer-reviewed publication of recent research.

American Running and Fitness Association

4405 East West Highway, Suite 405

Bethesda, MD 20814

Phone: (301) 913-9517

Fax: (301) 913-9520

E-mail: ARFARun@aol.com

This nonprofit, educational organization of athletes and sports medicine professionals distributes brochures and other information to the public about training, nutrition, and injury treatment and prevention. Members receive a monthly newsletter, *Running & FitNews*.

Road Runners Club of America

1150 South Washington Street, Suite 250

Arlington, VA 22314

Phone: (703) 836-0558

Fax: (703) 836-4430

E-mail: office@rrca.org

This nonprofit association consists of running club members. The national office provides services and information about running to local clubs and the general public. In addition to its quarterly magazine, *Footnotes*, it also produces brochures on children's running and other topics.

USA Track & Field

P.O. Box 120

Indianapolis, IN 46206

Phone: (317) 261-0500

Fax: (317) 261-0481

This organization is the national governing body for track and field, road racing, and racewalking in the United States. Its various committees and local associations administer running events and regulations. It also maintains race records, including age-group rankings.

Magazines and Newsletters

American Track and Field

Shooting Star Media

583 D'Onofrio Drive, Suite 203

Madison, WI 53719

Phone: (608) 827-0806

Fax: (608) 827-0811

This quarterly magazine focuses on competitive track and field. It's a good read for serious high school runners.

Race Results Weekly

P.O. Box 7388

FDR Station

New York, NY 10150

Phone: (212) 426-1228

Fax: (212) 426-2259

E-mail: rrweekly@juno.com

This weekly newsletter delivers open and age-group results of races throughout the world, as well as frequent news updates throughout the week. It's sent to subscribers by e-mail or fax by Monday morning, just 24 hours after most events are held.

Running & FitNews

4405 East West Highway, Suite 405

Bethesda, MD 20814

Phone: (301) 913-9517

Fax: (301) 913-9520

E-mail: ARFARun@aol.com

This monthly eight-page newsletter is published by the American Running and Fitness Association. It reports recent advances in sports medicine, exercise science, and nutrition, with an eye toward applying the findings to recreational runners' training. All of the articles are reviewed by an editorial board of sports medicine professionals.

Running, Ranting, Racing

7327 Green Oak Terrace

Lanham, MD 20706

E-mail: dsmn32a@prodigy.com

This monthly newsletter contains race reports and opinion pieces on the state of American running. It's written from an insider's point of view and is irreverent, satirical, and amusing.

Running Research News

P.O. Box 27041

Lansing, MI 48131

Phone: (517) 371-4897

Fax: (517) 371-4447

This newsletter comes out six times a year. It reports on recent exercise science research and shows how to apply these findings to your running. Its primary audience is serious road racers.

Running Times

98 N. Washington Street

Boston, MA 02114

Phone: (617) 367-2228

Fax: (617) 367-2350

E-mail: RTBakoulis@aol.com

This magazine contains training, nutrition, and sports medicine advice, shoe and apparel reviews, an extensive race calendar, profiles of today's runners, and commentary on running issues. It comes out 10 times a year. Bill Rodgers is a contributing editor.

Runner's World

33 East Minor Street

Emmaus, PA 18098

Phone: (610) 967-5171

Fax: (610) 967-8883

E-mail: rwedit@rodalepress.com

This monthly magazine is the largest running publication in the world. It's aimed primarily at beginning and intermediate runners. It contains articles on low-key training, cross-training, nutrition, and weight loss.

Footnotes

1150 South Washington Street, Suite 250

Arlington, VA 22314

Phone:(703) 836-0558

Fax: (703) 836-4430

E-mail: office@rrca.org

This quarterly magazine is the official publication of the Road Runners Club of America. It contains articles mostly of concern to grassroots runners, such as how to join and start a running club, book reviews, etc. RRCA members receive Footnotes as part of their membership.

Track and Field News

2570 El Camino Real, Suite 606

Mt. View, CA 94040

Phone: (415) 948-8188

Fax: (415) 948-9445

E-mail: edit@trackandfieldnews.com

This monthly magazine contains extensive coverage of track and field and cross-country at the high school through professional level.

The Internet

David Monti of *Race Results Weekly* assisted in compiling the following Web sites.

http://www.yahoo.com/Recreation/Sports/Running/

This site is the best starting point, listing more than 400 running-related Web sites.

http://www.runnersworld.com

This site provides news, race coverage, records, and training advice that's updated every working day.

http://www.coolrunning.com

Race results, stories, commentary, and race schedules are all available on this site.

http://www.doitsports.com

This site provides race results and race calendars.

http://www.usatf.org

This site is the home page of USATF, the national federation for road racing, track and field, and racewalking in the United States.

http://www.usaldr.org

This site provides long-distance running records, race courses, and USATF information.

http://tilastopaja.vservers.com

This site is a listing of track and field records and the year's top performances.

http://www.runningnetwork.com

You can find lots of regional magazines and results on this site.

http://sunsite.unc.edu/drears/running/running.html

This site is known as The Running Page and is a good site for recreational runners. It has many links.

http://rrca.org

This site is the home page of the Road Runners Club of America.

http://Fox.nstn.ca:80/~dblaikie/

This site is Ultramarathon World, the best site for information on races of 30 miles and longer.

http://www.geocities.com/Colosseum/7583/marguide.html

This site is The World Marathon Guide, with links to dozens of marathon pages.

http://www.kicksports.com/

This good general site has book reviews, race calendars, training advice, and a lot of links.

http://www.arfa.org

The home page of the American Running and Fitness Association includes articles on training, sports medicine, and nutrition, a listing of free running-related brochures, and help with choosing a running shoe.

The 100 Largest American Road Races in 1996

The following information is provided courtesy of USA Track & Field's Road Running Information Center.

Rank	Name	Distance	Location	Number of finishers
1	Lilac Bloomsday Run	12K	Spokane, WA	56,156
2	Examiner Bay to Breakers	12K	San Francisco, CA	53,030
3	Peachtree Road Race	10K	Atlanta, GA	50,000
4	Boston Marathon	26.2 miles	Boston, MA	35,868
5	Bolder Boulder	10K	Boulder, CO	34,782
6	New York City Marathon	26.2 miles	New York, NY	28,182
7	Honolulu Marathon	26.2 miles	Honolulu, HI	24,359
8	Race for the Cure	5K	Washington, DC	21,275
9	Crescent City Classic	10K	New Orleans, LA	20,000
10	Great Aloha Run	8.25 miles	Honolulu, HI	18,000
11	Office Depot Corporate Challenge	3.5 miles	Atlanta, GA	17,500
12	Chase Corporate Challenge	3.5 miles	New York, NY	16,500
13	Los Angeles Marathon	26.2 miles	Los Angeles, CA	16,180
14	Capitol 10,000	10K	Austin, TX	15,983
15	Quad-City Times Bix 7	7 miles	Davenport, IA	15,951
16	Revlon Run for Women	5K	Los Angeles, CA	15,314
17	Race for the Cure	5K	Portland, OR	15,283
18	Marine Corps Marathon	26.2 miles	Washington, DC	15,219

continues

Rank	Name	Distance	Location	Number of finishers
19	Office Depot Corporate Run	5K	Miami, FL	14,500
20	Chase Corporate Challenge	3.5 miles	Chicago, IL	14,022
21	Indianapolis Life 500 Festival	13.1 miles	Indianapolis, IN	12,969
22	Chase Corporate Challenge	3.5 miles	Boston, MA	12,000
23	Race for the Cure	5K	Peoria, IL	11,941
24	Cooper River Bridge Run	10K	Charleston, SC	11,454
25	Idaho Women's Fitness	5K	Boise, ID	11,200
26	St. Patrick's Day Dash	3.9 miles	Seattle, WA	11,000
27	Al's Walk	8K	Milwaukee, WI	10,501
28	Wharf to Wharf	10K	Capitola, CA	10,500
29	Chase Corporate Challenge	3.5 miles	New York, NY	10,000
30	Hood to Coast Relay	195 miles	Mt. Hood, OR	9,900
31	Race for the Cure	5K	New York, NY	9,200
32	Chicago Marathon	26.2 miles	Chicago, IL	9,196
33	Manchester Road Race	4.77 miles	Manchester, CT	9,070
34	Cowtown	10K	Ft. Worth, TX	9,069
35	Dallas YMCA Turkey Trot	3 miles	Dallas, TX	8,500
36	Chase Corporate Challenge	3.5 miles	Buffalo, NY	8,400
37	Junior Bloomsday	2 miles	Spokane, WA	8,100
38	Chase Corporate Challenge	3.5 miles	New York, NY	8,000
39	Race for the Cure	5K	Newport Beach, CA	7,885
40	Cherry Creek Sneak	5 miles	Denver, CO	7,777
41	Race for the Cure	5K	Detroit, MI	7,700
42	Army 10-Miler	10 miles	Washington, DC	7,579

Rank	Name	Distance	Location	Number of finishers
43	Race for the Cure	5K	Dallas, TX	7,421
44	Carlsbad 5000	5K	Carlsbad, CA	7,362
45	Race for the Cure	5K	Pittsburgh, PA	7,322
46	Omaha Corporate Cup	10K	Omaha, NE	7,295
47	Michael Forbes Trolley Run	4 miles	Kansas City, MO	6,905
48	Falmouth Road Race	7.1 miles	Falmouth, MA	6,851
49	Philadelphia Distance Run	13.1 miles	Philadelphia, PA	6,613
50	Race for the Cure	5K	Denver, CO	6,549
51	Gate River Run	15K	Jacksonville, FL	6,537
52	Portland to Coast Relay	126 miles	Portland, OR	6,500
53	Great Race	10K	Pittsburgh, PA	6,341
54	Sound to Narrows	12K	Tacoma, WA	6,285
55	Advil Mini Marathon	10K	New York, NY	6,153
56	Beach to Bay Relay	26.2 miles	Corpus Christi, TX	6,006
57	Race for the Cure	5K	Baltimore, MD	6,000
58	Run to the Far Side	5K	San Francisco, CA	5,900
59	Atlanta Half-Marathon	13.1 miles	Atlanta, GA	5,862
60	Revco-Cleveland	10K	Cleveland, OH	5,701
61	Spring Lake	5 miles	Spring Lake, NJ	5,700
62	Portland Marathon	26.2 miles	Portland, OR	5,587
63	Grandma's Marathon	26.2 miles	Duluth, MN	5,575
64	Utica Boilermaker	15K	Utica, NY	5,565
65	Gasparilla Distance Classic	15K	Tampa, FL	5,545
66	Twin Cities Marathon	26.2 miles	Minneapolis, MN	5,483
67	Shamrock Shuffle	8K	Chicago, IL	5,433
68	Race for the Cure	5K	Little Rock, AR	5,400
69	Dallas YMCA Turkey Trot	8 miles	Dallas, TX	5,200

continues

Rank	Name	Distance	Location	Number of finishers
70	Nortel Cherry Blossom	10 miles	Washington, DC	5,195
71	Get in Gear	10K	Minneapolis, MN	5,181
72	Gasparilla Distance Classic	5K	Tampa, FL	5,145
73	Crim Festival of Races	10 miles	Flint, MI	5,114
74	Race for the Cure	5K	Ft. Worth, TX	5,100
75	Race for the Cure	5K	Houston, TX	5,100
76	Chase Corporate Challenge	3.5 miles	Long Island, NY	5,100
77	Crazy Leggs	5 miles	Madison, WI	5,100
78	Race for Literacy	8K	San Diego, CA	4,929
79	America's Finest City	13.1 miles	San Diego, CA	4,825
80	Broad Street Run	10 miles	Philadelphia, PA	4,815
81	Celebration in the Oaks	2 miles	New Orleans, LA	4,800
82	Cannon Long Island	13.1 miles	East Meadow, NY	4,732
83	Kentucky Derby Festival	13.1 miles	Louisville, KY	4,714
84	Al's Run	8K	Milwaukee, WI	4,707
85	Bank IV River Run	2 miles	Wichita, KS	4,704
86	Chase Corporate Challenge	3.5 miles	Syracuse, NY	4,700
87	Redondo Beach Super Bowl	10K	Redondo Beach, CA	4,674
88	Race for the Cure	1.6 miles	Peoria, IL	4,600
89	Midnight Run	5 miles	New York, NY	4,500
90	Race for the Cure	5K	Memphis, TN	4,500
91	Beat the Bridge	8K	Seattle, WA	4,468
92	Race for the Cure	5K	San Francisco, CA	4,449
93	Dinosaur Dash	5K	Milwaukee, WI	4,388
94	Houston-Tenneco Marathon	26.2 miles	Houston, TX	4,347

Rank	Name	Distance	Number of Location	finishers
95	Tufts Run for Women	10K	Boston, MA	4,329
96	Azalea Trail Run	2 miles	Mobile, AL	4,300
97	New Times Phoenix	10K	Phoenix, AZ	4,300
98	Thanksgiving Turkey Trot	10K	Detroit, MI	4,300
99	Mercury News	10K	San Jose, CA	4,298
100	Race for the Cure	1 mile	Dallas, TX	4,263

Glossary

acclimatization   Getting used to running in the heat. It usually takes at least a few weeks.

aerobic exercise   An activity, such as running, that you do at a steady level of effort for at least 20 minutes at a time and during which you're never completely out of breath.

all comers' meet   A track meet at which runners of all levels of ability are welcome to participate.

amenorrhea   The absence of menstrual periods.

anti-inflammatories   Drugs that reduce swelling. Runners often take them when battling an injury.

ballistic stretching   Stretching that involves bouncing and sudden, jerking motions. It's the wrong way to stretch.

bandit   A runner who participates in a race without paying the registration fee.

biomechanics   How your body parts, especially your feet, work together to create your running form.

body composition   How much fat you carry compared to how much of your weight is comprised of lean material (muscles, bones, ligaments, and so on).

carbohydrates   Sugars and starches from your diet. Carbohydrates are your main source of energy when you run.

carboloading   Eating more carbohydrates than usual in the few days before a long race to boost your fuel stores.

cool-down   A short, slow jog after a race or hard run that helps you to recover more quickly.

CoolMax®   A fiber used in many running clothes that feels as soft as cotton but that keeps you more comfortable by not absorbing as much water.

course record   The fastest time run by anyone over a given race course.

cross-country race   A race that's held over grass and dirt.

cross-training   Doing other forms of aerobic exercise to supplement your running.

DNF   Stands for "did not finish." It describes a runner who drops out of a race.

doubling   Running twice in one day or running two races in a track meet.

fartlek   A Swedish word meaning "speed play." It's an unstructured form of speed work that you do on roads or trails rather than on a track.

fast-twitch fiber   A muscle fiber that powers explosive actions, such as sprinting, but that tires quickly.

flexibility   The ability to move your body through a full range of motion.

fun run   An untimed, low-key run, often only a mile long, usually held as part of a longer race.

glycogen   The substance carbohydrates are turned into when they are stored in your muscles. It's your body's preferred fuel source during aerobic exercise.

Heartbreak Hill   The last of the four hills between the 16- and 21-mile marks of the Boston Marathon.

heel counter   The back part of a running shoe that helps to make it more stable.

iliotibial band   A thick band of tissue that runs from your hip along your thigh to the outside of your knee.

insole   The removable inner part of a running shoe that provides cushioning and offers arch support.

intervals   Short runs, usually from a quarter-mile to one mile in length, that you run at faster than race pace to prepare for races.

junk miles   Miles that have no training purpose except to make your training log look more impressive.

kick   The all-out sprint that you do in the last few hundred yards of a race.

lactate threshold   The running speed at which your body can no longer clear lactate (a by-product of carbohydrate metabolism) from your blood as quickly as it produces it.

ladder   A speed workout in which the intervals increase and decrease in length.

layering   Wearing light layers of clothing during cold-weather running to trap body heat.

long run   A run that's at least one and a half times longer than any other run that you do in a week.

marathon   A race that is 26.2 miles long.

masters runner   A runner age 40 or older.

maximum heart rate   The greatest number of times that your heart can beat in a minute.

medial post   A firm section in the inner heel of a running shoe that increases the shoe's stability.

midsole   The part of a running shoe between the upper and outsole that provides most of the shoe's cushioning.

negative splits   Running the second half of a race faster than the first half.

orthotics   Devices placed in running shoes that help to prevent injury by fixing biomechanical problems.

outsole   The part of a running shoe that hits the ground and provides traction.

overpronation   When your feet roll in too much when you run. Overpronation is one of the leading causes of injury in runners.

overtraining   Running more than your body is prepared to for at least a few consecutive weeks. Overtraining can lead to injury and staleness.

overuse injuries   Injuries that result from repeatedly subjecting a body part to more force than it's prepared to handle. Most running injuries are overuse injuries.

oxygen debt   When you run so fast that your body needs more oxygen than you can take in. When you go into oxygen debt, you have to slow down.

plantar fasciitis   Inflammation of the plantar fascia, a thick band of fibrous tissue that runs along the bottom of your foot from your heel to your arch.

PR   Stands for "personal record," your fastest time for a given distance.

quarters   Intervals that are one-quarter mile long or one lap around a standard outdoor track.

resting heart rate   The number of times that your heart beats in one minute when you're still.

Runner's World   The world's most popular running magazine.

singlet   A tank top worn by runners in hot weather and during races.

splits   Your times at mile markers or other signposts along the way to the finish of a race.

speed work   Mixing short, fast runs with slow recovery jogs to prepare for races.

static stretching   Stretching that involves gradually lengthening muscles by holding the stretch for several seconds. Static stretching is the right way for runners to stretch.

striders   Runs of 100 yards or so that you do at near full speed to develop quickness and improve your form.

supination   When your feet don't roll in enough after they've hit the ground when you run.

talk test   Seeing whether you're able to carry on a conversation while you're running. If you can't pass the talk test on most runs, then you're running too quickly.

tapering   Reducing your mileage in the several days before an important race to gear up for a peak performance.

tempo run   A run of 20 to 40 minutes at your lactate threshold that you do to boost your performance in long races.

The Wall   What you crash into in a marathon, usually around 20 miles, when your body runs out of glycogen. When you hit The Wall, you have to slow down drastically.

training log   A written record of your training that helps you to monitor your progress and learn from your mistakes.

training partner   A runner of similar ability with whom you run at least occasionally.

tune-up races   Short races run as part of your preparation for longer, more important races.

ultramarathon   A race that's longer than a marathon. The most common ultramarathon is 50 miles.

upper   The top part of a running shoe that holds the laces.

VO_2 max   Scientific shorthand for maximum oxygen uptake, a measure of how much of the oxygen that you breathe while running your body can use. The higher your VO_2 max, the faster you can run.

warm-up   A short, easy jog before a race or hard run that prepares you for more intense activity.

wicking   The ability of a fiber to move moisture from your skin to the surface of a garment so that you stay more comfortable while running.

Index